Handbook of Cosmetic Skin Care

Handbook of Cosmetic Skin Care

Avi Shai, MD
Department of Dermatology, Soroka University Medical Center, Ben-Gurion University, Beer-Sheva, Israel

Howard I Maibach, MD
Department of Dermatology, University of California at San Francisco School of Medicine, San Francisco, USA

Robert Baran, MD
Nail Disease Center, Cannes, France

Line illustrations provided by Michal Yerushalmi-Rahamim

MARTIN DUNITZ

© Martin Dunitz Ltd 2001

First published in the United Kingdom in 2001

Paperback edition with corrections published in the United Kingdom in 2002 by
Martin Dunitz Ltd
The Livery House
7–9 Pratt Street
London NW1 0AE

Tel: +44(0) 20-7482-2202
Tel: +44(0) 20-7267-0159
E-mail: info.dunitz@tandf.co.uk
Website: http://www.dunitz.co.uk

A CIP catalogue record for this book is available from the British Library

ISBN 1-85317-752-0 hardback edition
ISBN 1-84184-179-X paperback edition, with corrections

Distributed in the USA by
Fulfilment Center
Taylor & Francis
7625 Empire Drive
Florence, KY 41042, USA
Toll Free Tel.: +1 800 634 7064
E-mail: cserve@routledge_ny.com

Distributed in Canada by
Taylor & Francis
74 Rolark Drive
Scarborough, Ontario M1R 4G2, Canada
Toll Free Tel.: +1 877 226 2237
E-mail: tal_fran@istar.ca

Distributed in the rest of the world by
Thomson Publishing Services
Cheriton House
North Way
Andover, Hampshire SP10 5BE, UK
Tel.: +44 (0) 1264 332424
E-mail: salesorder.tandf@thomsonpublishingservices.co.uk

Cover image: The Birth of Venus (detail). Sandro Botticelli (1444/5-1510).
Galleria degli Uffizi, Florence, Italy/Bridgeman Art Library.

Composition by Scribe, Gillingham, Kent, UK
Printed and bound in Singapore by Kyodo Printing pte Ltd.

Contents

Notes for the reader

In this book we have attempted to give a clear and easily understandable review of the topics presented, whilst maintaining a purely scientific approach, conforming to data supported by scientifically researched criteria. The book therefore relies on common, accepted knowledge in the field of dermatology, as it appears in the conventional dermatology textbooks and peer reviewed journals (such as those cited on Medline (PubMed), a computerized database of medical journal articles).

Sections of the text are highlighted in boxes – these present a more detailed explanation and discussion of some of the topics, and are intended for the more advanced reader.

Readers are advised to read first the introductory chapter on skin structure. In this chapter there are definitions of several basic terms such as 'epidermis' and 'dermis', which are used throughout the book.

Many of the chapters discuss common skin problems and conventional skin treatments, such as bleaching of dark skin spots and 'peeling'. These chapters are intended to broaden the reader's knowledge regarding the wide range of available regimens, not to encourage readers to diagnose and treat skin disorders requiring the advice of a dermatologist.

Contributors

Principles of Preparations of Medical and Cosmetic Products

Sima Halevy, MD
Professor of Dermatology
Ben-Gurion University
Chairman, Department of
Dermatology
Soroka University Medical Center
Beer Sheba
Israel

(with Avi Shai, MD)

Facial Cleansing Masks; Chemical Skin Peeling

Josef Shiri, MD
Senior Dermatologist
Chairman, Tel Aviv Institute of
Dermatology
General Health Fund
and Sheba Medical Center
Tel Hashomer
Tel Aviv
Israel

Acne; Liposomes

Alex Zvulunov, MD
Senior Lecturer, Ben Gurion
University
Senior Paediatrician and
Dermatologist
Chairman, Department of Paediatrics
Joseftal Hospital
Eilat
Israel

Sun and the Skin

Dafna Halle-Halevy, MD
Senior Dermatologist
Department of Dermatology
Soroka University Medical Center
Beer Sheba
Israel

Network of Blood Vessels on the Skin; Laser Treatment in Dermatology: Cosmetic Applications

Moshe Lapidoth, MD
Senior Dermatologist
Head of Laser Center
Rabin Medical Center
Petah Tikva
Israel

Cellulite; Alpha-hydroxy Acids

Ron Yaniv, MD
Senior Dermatologist
Sheba Medical Center
Tel Hashomer
Israel

Inflammation, Dermatitis and Cosmetics

Arieh Ingber, MD
Professor of Dermatology
The Hebrew University
Chairman, Department of
Dermatology
Hadassah Medical Center
Jerusalem
Israel

(with Avi Shai, MD)

Skin Tumours

Daniel Vardy, MD
Senior Lecturer
Ben-Gurion University
Senior Dermatologist
Chairman, Southern Region
Institute of Dermatology
General Health Fund
Beer Sheba
Israel

(with Avi Shai, MD)

*Active Ingredients in Cosmetic
Preparations*

Gil Yosipovitch, MD
Consultant Dermatologist
National Skin Center
Singapore 308205

Preparations used in Dermatology

Marcelo H Grunwald, MD
Senior Lecturer, Ben-Gurion
University
Senior Dermatologist
Department of Dermatology
Soroka University Medical Center
Beer Sheba
Israel

*Camouflaging Skin Lesions and
Other Disfiguring Conditions*

Victoria L Rayner
Dermatology Associate
University of California
Director of Training
Center of Appearance & Esteem
Training Institute
50 California Street, Suite 1500
San Francisco, California 9411
USA

*Structure of Hair and Principles of
Hair Care*

Emmilia Hodak, MD
Senior Lecturer, Tel Aviv University
Senior Dermatologist
Department of Dermatology
Rabin Medical Center
Petah Tikva
Israel

Hair Conditioners

Itzchak Shelkovitz-Shilo, MD
Senior Dermatologist
Sheba Medical Center
Tel Hashomer
Israel

*Methods for Temporary Removal of
Hair; Permanent Hair Removal:
Electrolysis – Electric Needle*

Zehava Laver, MD, PhD
Senior Dermatologist
General Health Fund
Tel Nordau
Tel Aviv
Israel

The Nails

Marina Landau, MD
Senior Dermatologist
Department of Dermatology
Ichilov Medical Center
Tel Aviv
Israel

(with Robert Baran, MD)

Acknowledgements

The authors wish to thank the following for their valuable help and contribution to this text: Audra J Geras and Novartis for the illustrations on pages 6, 10, 11, 103 and 151; Dr L Kachko for the figures on pages 12, 13 and 66; Professor Axel Hoke for the figure on page 123 and 125 (left); Nikolaus J Smeh for the figures on pages 171, 172 and 173, which are taken from his book, *Creating Your Own Cosmetics – Naturally* (Alliance Publishing House, 1995); R N Richards, MD and G E Meharg, RN for the figures on pages 286, 294 (right), 297, 298 and 299, which are taken from their book, *Cosmetic and Medical Electrolysis and Temporary Hair Removal: A Practice Manual and Reference Guide*, Second edition (Medric Limited, 1997); Dr Emanuela Cagnano for the figures on pages 7 and 107; Dr Marcelo H Grunwald for the figure on page 159 (bottom right); Dr Bernardo Mosovich for the figure on page 154; Professor Amiram Sagi for the figure on page 159 (upper right); the following contributors to *Textbook of Cosmetic Dermatology*, 2nd edition (Martin Dunitz, 1998) who have kindly allowed their material to be used: Dr A A Ramelet (two illustrations on page 124); Dr Timothy J Rosio (four illustrations on page 236); Dr Rodney Dawber (two illustrations on page 275); Professor Ronald Marks for the illustrations on page 153 (middle) and 156 (right), which are taken from his book, *Skin Disease in Old Age*, 2nd edition (Martin Dunitz, 1999); Janssen Pharmaceutica for the illustration on page 271; Mosby Inc for the illustrations on page 182 (reproduced from Olsen EA et al, Tretinoin emollient cream: A new therapy for photodamaged skin. *J Am Acad Derm* 1992; **26**: 215–24); on page 191 (reproduced from Ditre CM et al, Effects of α-hydroxy acids on photoaged skin: A pilot clinical, histologic, and ultrastructured study. *J Am Acad Derm* 1996; **34**: 187-95); and on page 192 (reproduced from Bergfeld W et al, Improving the cosmetic appearance of photoaged skin with glycolic acid. *J Am Acad Derm* 1997; **36**: 1011–13).

Finally, our particular thanks to Dr Gary Zentner for assistance with editing and preparation of the text; to Dr Gil Yosipovitch for his initiative in this project; to Professor Reuven Bergman, Professor Sima Halevy and Professor Michael David for reviewing chapters in the book; to Dr Alex Zvulunov for his assistance and for his contribution stemming from a broad knowledge in medicine and dermatology; and to Mr Naftali Oron for his most valuable ongoing advice throughout the course of this project.

1

Cosmetics and cosmetic preparations: Basic definitions

Contents Basic definitions • Definition of a cosmetic product • Classification of cosmetic preparations • The grey area between a drug and a cosmetic product

Basic definitions

Cosmetics deals with those aspects of the skin related to beauty. This profession concentrates on skin care, protecting the skin, and improving its appearance. 'Cosmetic' is derived from the Greek *kosmesis* (adorning), from *kosmeo* (to order or arrange).

A **cosmetician** is a person who is engaged in the field of cosmetics, whose work is directed towards the care, protection and improvement in appearance of the skin.

Dermatology refers to the medical specialty dealing with the diagnosis and treatment of skin, hair and nail diseases.

A **dermatologist** is a doctor who is trained and experienced in the various aspects of skin disease. Dermatologists are supposed to know best all about skin care, protecting the skin and its health.

The term **cosmetology** is relatively vague, and cannot always be found in dictionaries. It refers to the scientific and investigative basis of cosmetics, in its biological, chemical and medical ramifications.

The term **cosmetologist** is derived from the term 'cosmetology'. In its broad meaning, it refers to someone who specializes in the investigative aspects of cosmetics: he/she can be a chemist, a biologist or a physician. However, this definition varies from one country to another. In some countries, such as the USA, it is a formal title subjected to the regulations of each state, to obtain which one has to graduate from a school of cosmetics. In other countries, there is no recognized medical/professional specialty of cosmetology, so, in practice, the title of 'cosmetologist' may be abused by anyone who decides to call himself/herself as such.

Definition of a cosmetic product

The US Food, Drug and Cosmetic (FDC) Act defines cosmetics as:

'(1)   articles intended to be rubbed, poured, sprinkled or sprayed on, introduced into, or otherwise applied to the human body or any part thereof for cleansing, beautifying, promoting attractiveness, or altering the appearance; and
(2)   articles intended for use as a component of any such articles except that such a term shall not include soap.'

There is a significant difference between cosmetic products and drugs (including drugs intended for application to the skin), which the reader should be familiar with. Drugs are defined in the FDC Act as including:

'articles intended for use in the diagnosis, cure, mitigation, treatment or prevention of disease in man ... articles (other than food) intended to affect the structure or any function of the body of man.'

It follows from the above that a cosmetic product (not being a drug) is not meant to affect the structure or function of the skin. However, as will be discussed below, nowadays this 'strict' definition is becoming more and more blurred.

Classification of cosmetic preparations

Cosmetic preparations are classified in accordance with their function:

- those that improve appearance and beautify
- those related to skin care
- those related to skin protection

Improving appearance and beautifying
The aim is to produce a pleasant, attractive appearance, by emphasizing those areas of the face or body that look better, so as to focus the observer's gaze on them. At the same time, an attempt is made to camouflage and correct skin lesions, if necessary. This category of cosmetic products includes various make-ups, hair dyes, nail polish, etc.

Skin care
Cosmetics are used to try and obtain (and retain) a smooth, soft supple skin. Moisturizing and cleansing preparations belong to this category (some have a protective effect). Those preparations said to 'prevent ageing' are also rightly classified in this category.

Skin protection

The aim is to protect the skin from the external effects of the sun, wind, cold, etc. Sunscreen preparations belong to this category. Moisturizers also have a protective effect on the skin. Soaps that contain antibacterial substances are also included in this category, since they do provide a certain degree of antibacterial protection to the skin.

The grey area between a drug and a cosmetic product

In the past, the division between cosmetic products and drugs was clear-cut. Nearly all cosmetics were no more (and did not usually claim to be anything other) than simple moisturizing, cleansing or colouring products.

Currently, the boundary between drugs and cosmetic products for skin care is becoming blurred. Many cosmetic products are marketed with statements such as:

- 'Accelerates the renewal of cells'
- 'Builds up supportive tissue in the skin'
- 'Repairs sun damage to the skin'
- 'Repairs skin ageing'

It is obvious that all of the above effects can be achieved only by drugs, since they relate to changes in the function and structure of the tissue.

Sometimes the difference between a cosmetic product and a drug lies in the concentration of the active ingredient in the product. For example, in low concentrations, alpha-hydroxy acids function essentially as moisturizing agents; it is only at higher concentrations that they have any significant effect on the epidermis.

Not only is the border between cosmetic products and drugs fuzzy, but there is also a grey area between cosmetic treatments and dermatology. A cosmetician's treatment can certainly alter the structure and function of the skin – for example in the treatment of acne, in the application of 'permanent' make-up, etc.

Therefore some modern cosmetic products lie in an increasingly grey area, and can almost be defined as medications. This fact confers a serious responsibility on those involved in cosmetic treatment, requiring them to have a fairly deep knowledge of the subject, and to exercise careful judgement, thoughtful deliberation and maximum care when using the cosmetic products at their disposal.

2
Skin structure

Contents Overview • Thickness of the skin • Functions of the skin • The outer layer: epidermis • Dermis • Sub-cutis: the layer of fat beneath the dermis

Overview

Familiarity with the structure and function of the skin is essential for a clear understanding of all the chapters in this book.

- **Epidermis** – the outer layer. At the base of this layer, the cells are continuously dividing, forming new cells. As cells are made, they are pushed towards the surface by the newer cells underneath them, and eventually reach the keratinous layer. Finally, the outermost cells in the keratinous layer are shed.
- **Dermis** – the layer below the epidermis is thicker than the latter. The dermis is made up mainly of collagen and elastin fibres. It contains blood vessels, nerves, sensory organs, sebaceous glands, sweat glands and the hair follicles.
- **Sub-cutis** – this layer lies beneath the dermis, and consists of fat cells.

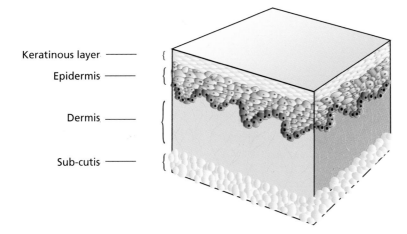

Keratinous layer
Epidermis
Dermis
Sub-cutis

Structure of the skin.

The diagram on the previous page is important; keep it in mind, since it will be referred to throughout the book. We shall discuss each layer in detail.

Thickness of the skin

The thickness of the skin ranges from 1 mm to 4 mm. This thickness, and those of each of its layers, vary in different areas.

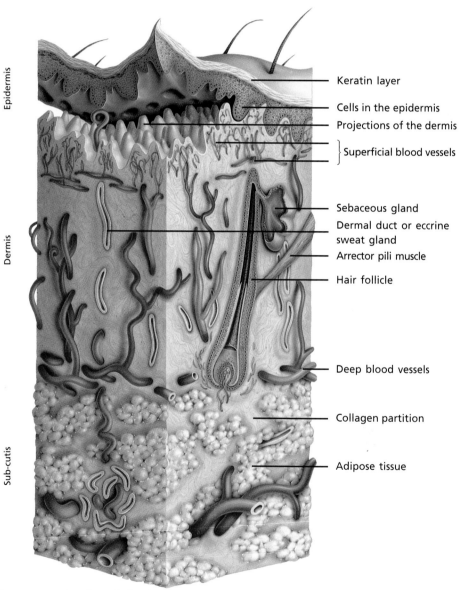

Transverse section through the skin.

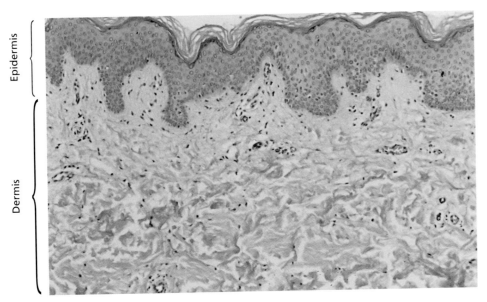

Epidermis

Dermis

Skin structure viewed through a microscope lens.

The epidermis is generally thin. It is particularly so in the skin of the eyelids: approximately 0.1 mm. The epidermis is particularly thick in the areas of the soles and palms, where it is about 1 mm deep.

The dermis is up to 20 times as thick as the epidermis. It tends to be particularly thick on the back, where it can reach a thickness of approximately 3–4 mm.

There is also variability in the thickness of the sub-cutis skin layer, which tends to be thicker in the thigh and abdominal areas, and particularly thin in the face.

Functions of the skin

The skin has the following functions:

- it acts as a protective layer
- it transmits sensations
- it helps to regulate the body's temperature
- it produces vitamin D
- it plays a role in social interactions

Protective layer
The skin serves as a covering that protects the body from:

- mechanical damage such as that caused by friction, different levels of pressure and various kinds of impact;

- chemical toxins – the outermost layer of the skin is made of a tough keratin that can withstand (to a certain extent) various toxic substances such as acids;
- ultraviolet rays from the sun;
- infectious agents such as bacteria and fungi – the skin is continuously exposed to bacteria, but the tightly packed structure of the cells in the keratin layer renders it relatively impermeable and thereby prevents bacteria from penetrating the skin.

Bacteria and fungi

There are always many bacteria on the skin surface, but these usually cause no harm. Provided the skin is normal and healthy, and the keratin layer is intact, these bacteria cannot penetrate and enter the skin. As a rule, most bacteria found in the human body are not pathogenic, i.e. they do not cause disease. However, any damage to the skin, be it a burn, a wound, or any other damage, can result in bacteria invading the skin and causing an infection.

In contrast to bacteria, certain types of fungi can infiltrate and damage the integrity of keratin; this explains why fungal skin infections are more common than bacterial infections. Furthermore, once the fungi have damaged the skin's integrity, it is easier for bacteria to invade the skin, so it is common for bacterial infections to occur in skin already infected by a fungus.

The skin serves not only to protect the body from the external environment; another important function of the skin is to prevent loss of water from the body. If it were not for this important property of the skin, the body would lose substantial amounts of water, to an extent that would threaten life. The importance of this function can be seen in patients whose skin has been damaged, for example by widespread burns. These patients suffer enormous fluid losses, and initial resuscitation must always include the provision of large volumes of fluids.

Transmission of sensations
The dermis is richly supplied with nerves, which transmit sensations of touch, pressure, pain and temperature from the skin.

Temperature regulation
As water on the surface of the skin evaporates, it has a cooling effect and lowers the body temperature. The same applies to sweat as it evaporates. The amount of sweat released from the skin varies depending on the body temperature and the environmental conditions, and may reach several litres per day.

The body temperature is regulated by alterations in the amount of blood flowing to the skin, and in the evaporation of water.

Production of vitamin D

Exposure to sunlight stimulates the production of vitamin D in the skin. The vitamin then passes from the skin into the blood, and reaches the various tissues of the body where it exerts its effects. Vitamin D is essential for the regulation of calcium levels in the body, and for the structure and growth of the bones.

Social interaction

The skin – through its colour, its texture and its smell – 'transmits' sexual and social messages. Thus blushing, resulting from dilatation of the blood vessels in the skin, reflects embarrassment; facial expressions reflect various emotions, etc.

The outer layer: epidermis

Epidermis; keratinocytes

The epidermis is the outermost layer of the skin. This layer is made up of approximately 15–20 tightly packed layers of cells. Most of the cells in this layer are **keratinocytes**, or **squamous cells** (Latin: *squama* = scale). Each cell is a few thousandths of a millimetre in size.

As seen in the figure below, the lowermost layer of the epidermis is the **basal layer**, obviously called such because the cells that comprise it form the base of the epidermis.

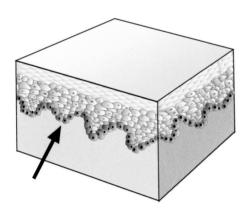

The basal layer of the epidermis.

In the basal layer, new epidermal cells are formed by cell division. The skin cells formed in the basal layer are pushed upwards by 'younger' cells, until they are ultimately shed from the surface of the skin. This is a continuous process. Every moment of our lives, without our being aware of it, our skin is renewing itself as millions of cells slowly move outward.

As the cells move upwards, their shape becomes flatter and flatter. As they move, they start to degenerate, and gradually lose their vitality. They lose their water content, dry out, and flatten out. By the time they reach the outermost layers, the cells are dead.

The outermost layer of the skin is the **keratinous (horny) layer** (Greek: *keras* = horn). There the cells are dead, flattened, and lie closely packed on each other like roof tiles. The cells of the outer layers contain large quantities of a protein called **keratin.**

From the time a new cell forms in the basal layer until it is shed from the surface of the skin takes approximately 28 days. This means that most cells of the skin are replaced by new ones every 28 days.

The keratinous layer is made of tightly packed dead cells, which gives the skin the protective capabilities listed above.

Increased turnover of cells in the epidermis

In various diseases (such as psoriasis or seborrhoeic dermatitis), there is an increase in the turnover of cells in the skin, so keratin accumulates abnormally on the skin's surface. This takes the form of thick scales or flakes on the skin.

Other epidermal cells: Langerhans cells, melanocytes

In addition to the keratinocytes, which are the basic cells of the epidermis, there are also other types of cells: **Langerhans cells** and **melanocytes.**

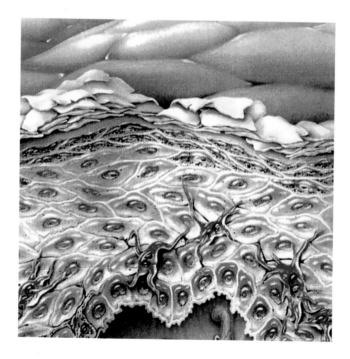

Melanocytes (shown in red) scattered throughout the cells of the epidermis.

Langerhans cells
These are involved in the body's immune system.

Melanocytes
These cells produce a pigment called **melanin**, which gives the skin its dark colour. The melanin produced by melanocytes is passed on to the keratinocytes.

   Approximately one in ten cells in the basal layer of the epidermis is a melanocyte. The differences in skin colour between different individuals and between races are determined genetically by the amount of melanin produced by the melanocytes and its distribution throughout the skin. In fact, differences in skin shade and colour are determined not by the number and density of the melanocytes, which are basically identical in all humans of any race, but by their degree of activity.

   Exposure to sunlight stimulates the production of melanin.

Dermis

The dermis lies beneath the epidermis. Its upper level has projections that extend into corresponding depressions in the epidermis.

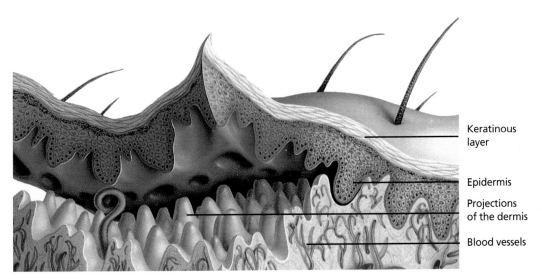

Keratinous layer

Epidermis

Projections of the dermis

Blood vessels

Schematic representation of the wave-like junction between the epidermis and the dermis, with corresponding projections and depressions.

   The dermis is mainly composed of an amorphous (i.e. without shape or structure) intercellular substance that acts as a sort of 'cement' for all the components of the dermis. Within this amorphic substance are:

• cells of the dermis

- collagen and elastin fibres
- blood vessels
- nerves and sensory organs
- sebaceous glands
- hairs
- sweat glands

Dermal cells

The basic cell of the dermis is the **fibroblast**. This cell produces the intercellular substance as well as collagen fibres.

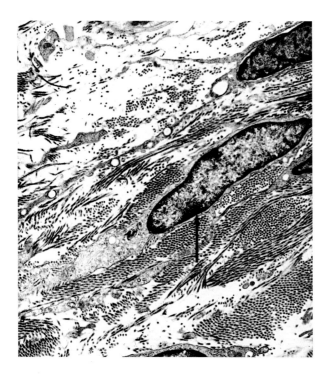

Fibroblast (indicated by the arrow) as seen under the electron microscope; the round-shaped bodies seen in this picture are collagen fibres as seen in transverse section.

Other cells within the dermis include **white blood cells (leukocytes)**, which are involved in defence against infections. Under normal circumstances, their number in the dermis is negligible. The number of leukocytes increases when there is inflammation or infection in the skin.

Collagen and elastin fibres

Collagen and **elastin** are proteins in the form of fibres. The fibres are intertwined throughout the intercellular substance, and provide the dermis with its strength and elasticity:

- The collagen fibres give the skin its strength.

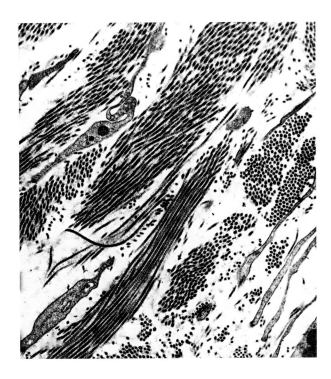

Collagen fibres as seen under the electron microscope.

- Elastin fibres are thinner than collagen fibres; they are responsible for the skin's elasticity – its ability to 'spring back' to its original form after being stretched.

If these fibres are damaged (as a result of ageing, or from excessive, cumulative exposure to the sun), the skin becomes loose, does not return to its original state when stretched, and looks thin and wrinkled.

Blood vessels in the dermis

The major function of the blood is to transport nutrients and oxygen to every organ in the body (including the skin), and to remove waste products and carbon dioxide produced in the various cells of the body. Note that there are no blood vessels in the epidermis. On the other hand, the dermis is richly endowed with blood vessels, and the epidermis receives its nutrients and oxygen directly from the dermis.

In the dermis, the blood vessels (which are continuations of larger vessels deeper in the body) branch out into smaller and smaller vessels that cover the entire area of the skin. Widening and narrowing (dilatation and constriction) of the blood vessels occur in response to changes in temperature, and form one of the most important mechanisms for controlling the body's temperature. Dilatation of the blood vessels results in the skin becoming pinker, or even red – as seen in blushing or when the temperature rises.

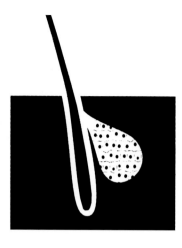

A hair follicle with its associated sebaceous gland.

Sebaceous glands

These glands are attached to the hair follicles, and their contents are secreted into the follicle through a tiny duct. The glands secrete **sebum** – a fatty substance that emerges from the opening of the hair follicle onto the skin surface and coats the skin with an oily layer.

Hair

Hair is present on every area of the body, except the palms and soles, the red areas of the lips, the skin over the knuckles, and the genital organs. Hair grows out of an elongated tubular structure in the skin called a **hair follicle**, as shown in the diagrams on page 15.

Each hair has an elongated part, which grows from the dermis and protrudes above the surface of the skin, known as the **shaft (or body) of the hair**. At the lower end of the hair follicle, there is a swelling, where the **hair root cells** are to be found. These cells have a striking capacity for replication. As they divide, the new cells so formed at the root of the hair are aligned vertically and move upwards; thus the hair grows longer and longer. As the cells move upwards, they die off – in the same way as do the skin cells in the epidermis (the keratinocytes) as they move up to the surface of the skin.

The upper part of the hair that protrudes above the skin surface is therefore composed of keratinous 'dead' matter. The main substance in the hair cells that died as they moved upwards is a special form of the protein keratin. The keratin in hair is hard, and is therefore called **'hard keratin'**, which differs in its chemical composition from the keratin of the horny layer of the skin.

The shaft of the hair is made up of a large number of thin, delicate, intertwined fibres. The main component of these fibres is, as noted above, keratin.

The structure and life cycle of hair is dealt with in more detail in Chapter 25.

Attached to the hairs are tiny muscles (**arrectores pilorum muscles**). When these muscles contract, the hair stands up. These muscles have nothing to do with the secretion of sebum. In some animals, the contraction of these muscles causes the fur to stand up – in response to danger, etc.; in the human, the sudden contraction of these muscles in a given area causes 'goose bumps'.

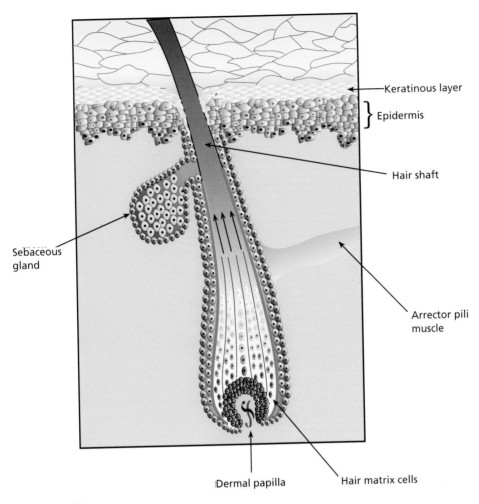

Keratinous layer

Epidermis

Hair shaft

Sebaceous gland

Arrector pili muscle

Dermal papilla

Hair matrix cells

Structure of hair.

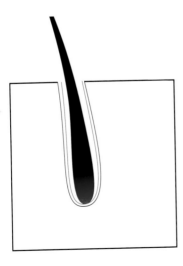

Schematic representation of a hair follicle (shown in red).

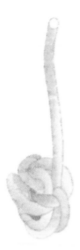

Eccrine sweat gland.

Eccrine sweat glands

An **eccrine sweat gland** is a long tube whose base, which is very convoluted, is in the lower part of the dermis. The tube passes all the way up through the dermis and the epidermis, and ends in a tiny sweat pore on the surface of the skin.

There are between two and three million eccrine sweat glands in the body, but they are not distributed evenly. There are more eccrine sweat glands in the areas of the face, the palms and the soles. The amount of sweat also varies considerably from day to day, but can reach several litres in a day.

The main function of the sweat glands is to regulate body temperature. As sweat evaporates from the surface of the skin, it lowers the skin temperature, with a subsequent decrease in the body's temperature.

The secretion of the sweat is controlled through nerve endings attached to sweat glands. Physical effort, warm weather, fever or emotional stress stimulate the sweat glands, which secrete sweat. Sweat is largely water, with small amounts of salts. Usually, the sweat secreted by eccrine sweat glands does not cause body odour.

Apocrine sweat glands

These glands, unlike the eccrine sweat glands, are not distributed on most of the skin surface. They are larger and more convoluted than the eccrine sweat glands, and are found mainly:

- in the armpits
- in the genital area
- around the nipples

Similar glands are present in the external ear canals and the eyelids. These sweat glands are present at birth, but only develop and start to secrete during adolescence. They have no obvious physiological function in humans. In other mammals, the apocrine glands produce an odour involved in sexual attraction.

The secretion from the apocrine glands is relatively thick and has a 'milky' consistency. This secretion is responsible for the formation of unpleasant body odour. In the form in which it is secreted, it has no smell; however, subsequently, the organic compounds in it are broken down by bacteria, and the products of this breakdown are characterized by an unpleasant smell.

Sub-cutis: the layer of fat beneath the dermis

This layer of fat acts as a cushioning layer to protect vital inner organs from mechanical trauma, and also as an insulating layer to protect against cold. In addition, the fat is an important energy store for the body.

The amount and distribution of the fat depends largely on hereditary factors, on diet and on physical activity.

Groups of fat cells are separated by rigid partitions made up mainly of collagen fibres, as illustrated in the figure.

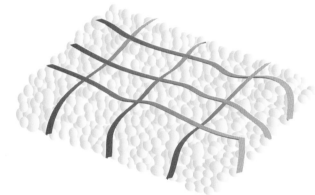

Groups of fat cells separated by collagen partitions.

3

Principles of preparation of medical and cosmetic products

Contents Overview • Bases in cosmetic and medical products – fatty bases • Bases in cosmetic and medical products – water, aqueous solutions • Bases in cosmetic and medical products – powders • Combinations of bases • Combining a fatty base with water • Types of cream • Combining a powder with water: suspensions • Combining a powder with a fatty base: pastes • Other combinations • Preservatives • Summary • Addendum: gels

Overview

This chapter reviews the principles of preparation of cosmetic products. The same principles used in the preparation of cosmetic products also apply to the preparation of medical compounds for the skin, except that the latter incorporate a medication or medications to treat some skin abnormality. Both cosmetic and medical preparations for application to the skin are called **preparations for external use**. A cosmetic or medical preparation for external use consists of three components:

- **active ingredient**
- **base** (or **vehicle**)
- **additional/auxiliary substances**

In neither cosmetic nor medical use is the active ingredient meant to be applied to the skin in its pure chemical form. In every case, the active ingredient is combined with a base, and with other substances, thereby creating the effective preparation. This combination ensures that the active ingredient penetrates into the skin.

Active ingredient
The active ingredient might be, for example:

- an antibiotic medication, used for the treatment of acne or a bacterial skin infection;
- an antifungal medication to treat a skin infection caused by a fungus;

- a substance intended to inhibit ageing of the skin (e.g. retinoic acid or an alpha-hydroxy acid);
- a substance that lightens dark lesions on the skin (e.g. hydroquinone).

The active ingredient is, in effect, the main component of the preparation for external use, and it is its action that produces the main effect of the preparation. However, as stated above, the active ingredient does not usually appear on its own. It must be incorporated into the base of the preparation.

Base (vehicle)

This is the material that 'carries' the active ingredient into the skin. It is called the 'base' or the 'vehicle', in the sense of transporting something, since it 'conveys' the active ingredient to the skin. The base must ensure that the active ingredient remains chemically stable, that it can penetrate the skin efficiently, and that it can be released effectively within the skin.

The three elemental bases are:

- fatty bases
- water, aqueous solutions
- powders

By using one of the above, or a combination of them, one can produce the wide array of bases used in dermatology and in the cosmetics industry: ointments, creams, emulsions, solutions, powders, pastes, suspensions or lotions.

Note that the role of the base in a cosmetic or dermatological preparation is not merely that of a wrapping around a medicine or an active ingredient in the preparation, or a vehicle that transports the active ingredient into the skin. In many cases, the base itself may have specific effects on the skin, such as increasing the moisture level, soothing or cooling, as will be described further on.

A considerable portion of the cosmetics industry is devoted to these bases alone, without the addition of any active ingredients.

Additional/auxiliary substances

Medicinal or cosmetic preparations usually also contain other substances. Common additives are:

- fragrances and perfumes
- coloured dyes
- preservatives

Preservatives in cosmetic preparations are discussed later in this chapter.

Bases in cosmetic and medical products – fatty bases

The main uses of fatty bases in dermatology and cosmetics are as follows:

- Fatty bases may enable medicines incorporated within them to better penetrate the skin.

- Fatty bases increase the skin's moisture level by creating an oily film on its surface, thus reducing the amount of water evaporating from the skin.

Fatty bases may be derived from animal sources, plant sources or mineral sources (the most common mineral source is crude oil, from which various oils can be derived after refining). In general, fatty bases from any of those sources can be in liquid, semi-solid or solid form. The terminology commonly used is as follows:

- a fatty base that appears in liquid form (at room temperature) is called an **oil**;
- a fatty base that appears in semi-solid form is called a **fat**;
- a fatty base that appears in solid form is called a **wax**.

The widely used terminology regarding fatty bases and the chemical definitions

The above definitions are those in everyday use, but are not strictly accurate in terms of the chemical definitions of oils, fats and waxes. Furthermore, it should be remembered that the chemical and cosmetics industries can alter the physical properties of fatty substances, and mix them with other substances. Thus, for example, a substance that was originally a liquid (oil) can appear in a semi-solid state as part of some compound.

Animal-derived fatty bases

Lanolin
This is a complex compound derived from sheep's wool. It is made from the oily substance secreted by the sheep's sebaceous glands, and is a basic ingredient in many moisturizing compounds. In its original, pure form, lanolin is a yellowish-grey, sticky substance with a characteristic smell. By various chemical and physical processes, a variety of substances can be derived from lanolin, with different properties: substances that are less sticky, odourless, of different shades, etc.

Since lanolin is fairly similar in composition to sebum, which is secreted by human sebaceous glands, it rarely causes irritation when applied to the skin. Nevertheless, skin sensitivity can occasionally occur due to lanolin or lanolin-based products.

Wool alcohols
These substances are also derived from sheep's wool. Chemically, wool alcohols contain more alcoholic oily compounds than does lanolin – a quality that enables these substances to contain more water in their composition.

Spermaceti
This is an oily substance produced by whales. Its use is prohibited in the USA. In view of the source of this oil, consumers who have reservations about the killing of whales may prefer not to use moisturizing preparations that contain this substance, and should check the details on the package of any moisturizer to ensure that it does not contain spermaceti. Synthetic spermaceti, on the other hand, is a chemically synthesized wax that can be used as a replacement for natural spermaceti.

Note: The way in which all these animal-derived oils act on the skin is identical. There is no significant difference in the cosmetic or medicinal value of the different substances. They have no effect in preventing ageing of the skin. There is no advantage in using oils derived from rarer animals, and their use is only an uncalled-for commercial gimmick. Mink oil, for example, produced from the skin of minks, or whale-derived oil have no advantage over lanolin in terms of their cosmetic or medicinal effects.

Plant-derived fatty bases: plant oils

There is a wide variety of oils derived from various plants, for example olive oil, sesame oil, peanut oil, corn oil, sunflower oil, soy oil and cocoa butter. The chemical composition of plant oils or animal-derived oils and the presence of saturated fatty acids or unsaturated fatty acids is significant when talking of diet and nutrition. However, it is of no relevance when we are talking about the external use of these oils: in terms of their cosmetic and dermatological effects, the efficacy of plant oils is similar to those that are animal-derived, and the ratio of polyunsaturated to saturated oils in their composition is irrelevant.

Fatty bases derived from minerals

This group includes the paraffin oils, which are products of the refining of crude oil. Substances derived from paraffin can be in a liquid, semi-solid or solid state:

- liquid paraffin (liquid petroleum)
- semi-solid paraffin, white soft paraffin (petroleum jelly, semi-solid petrolatum)
- wax is solid paraffin

The natural colour of paraffin is yellow, but it usually undergoes chemical bleaching processes. Paraffins are efficient occlusives and thus can prevent water evaporation from the skin. They are inert, so they very rarely cause skin irritation and sensitivity. However, they are not very convenient for day-to-day use, since they produce an unpleasant greasy feeling on the skin.

Notes

- For further details on the various cosmetic preparations that contain animal-, plant- or mineral-derived fatty bases, see Chapter 4 on skin moisture and moisturizers.
- In general, different fatty bases can be mixed together to achieve the desired properties.

What is an ointment?

An **ointment** is the accepted name for a preparation (medical or cosmetic) that is meant to be applied on the skin and whose base is composed of fatty substances; the fatty bases of the ointment produce the typical semi-solid consistency.

The fatty base may allow better skin penetration of the active ingredients incorporated within the ointment. Thus various medications can be incorporated into an ointment, thereby producing, for example, antibiotic ointments or corticosteroid ointments.

The 'classic' ointments, such as petroleum jelly, are based on fatty substances derived from minerals. Petroleum jelly is an inert, water-repellent substance that creates an occlusive layer on the skin. Fatty preparations derived from minerals (as compared with other types of skin preparations) are better occlusives, which protect the skin effectively, and also tend not to rinse off the skin readily.

Products based on fatty substances such as lanolin or eucerin can contain water. The addition of water to the oil makes the product more aesthetically pleasing; it is less sticky, more pleasant to the touch and easier to use.

As described below, when a tiny amount of water is added to a fatty base that is in a semi-solid state, it is still called an ointment; however, above a certain amount of water, the preparation becomes a **cream**.

Bases in cosmetic and medical products – water, aqueous solutions

The commonest liquid used in cosmetic preparations is water. Usually, in dermatology, water is not used on its own, but a medication or some other active ingredient is dissolved in water (in the same way as sugar or salt can be dissolved in water), thereby producing a solution. In solution, molecules of the dissolved substance spread equally and are evenly distributed in the water. Therefore a solution has a clear and uniform appearance.

Water can be combined with various forms of cosmetic substances. As discussed below, it can be mixed with oils or powders.

Furthermore, water has additional effects on the cooling and drying of the skin. Since water evaporates from the skin's surface, it has a cooling effect. As the water evaporates, it 'drags' with it additional water found in the outer layers of the skin – so wetting the skin frequently with water actually has a drying effect! As a result of this, in dermatology, when we want to dry out inflamed, weeping areas of skin, we do so by repeatedly wetting those areas.

Tincture – an alcohol-based solution

Alcohol can also be used in cosmetic preparations. Since alcohol evaporates faster than water, it has an even stronger cooling effect. Alcohol is also effective to some extent in killing bacteria. However, the higher the concentration of the alcohol, the more it tends to irritate the skin. An alcohol-based solution is called a **tincture**.

Bases in cosmetic and medical products – powders

In both the cosmetics industry and dermatology, use is made of fine powders that do not contain coarse particles. Powders are made of one or more solid ingredients. They are intended for application to healthy skin. The main purposes of powders are to:

- prevent friction
- absorb excess moisture

Powders are usually used in skin creases (such as the groin), since those are the areas where moisture tends to accumulate, and where friction occurs. In addition, in cosmetics, powders are used in many types of make-up preparations to cover and conceal certain areas of the skin.

Substances commonly used in powders

Among the substances used in powders are the following:

Zinc oxide has covering and protecting properties.

Titanium dioxide has protective properties against ultraviolet rays. It is a significant component of sunscreens.

Talc is actually the commercial name for **magnesium polysilicate**. Commercial preparations usually contain small amounts of other substances, such as zinc oxide or aluminium silicate. Talc is an inert substance that is effective in preventing friction.

Calamine is a mixture of zinc oxide with a small amount of iron oxide. It has a soothing effect on the skin, and can decrease itching to some extent.

Starch absorbs liquids effectively, and is therefore used in the treatment of excessively moist skin.

Note: In general, it is not advisable to use pure powders on babies, since, as the powder is being applied to the skin, the fine particles disperse into the air, and may be inhaled.

Combinations of bases

So far we have discussed each of the three elemental bases separately, namely fatty bases, water and aqueous solutions, and powders.

A combination of various bases in different preparations creates the extensive range of cosmetic and medicinal substances intended for application to the skin. This is usually illustrated using a coloured triangle, which shows how different combinations of the various bases can create a wide variety of preparations:

- combining a **fatty base and water** produces a **liquid emulsion** or **cream**;
- combining **powder and water** produces a **suspension**;
- combining a **fatty base** and **powder** produces a **paste**.

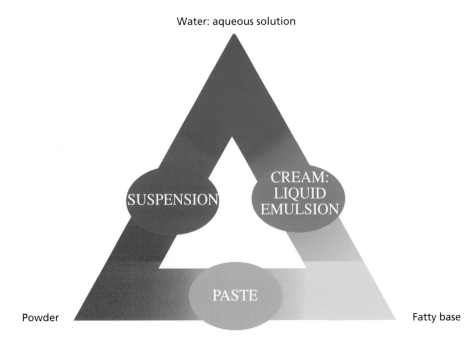

The triangle illustrating the various possibilities in combining bases.

Combining a fatty base with water

Mixing water and oil
What happens when water and oil are poured together into the same vessel? Since oil does not dissolve in water, the answer is simple: the oil floats on top of the water, since its specific gravity is less than that of water.

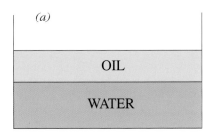

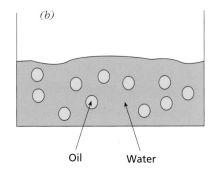

(a) Vessel containing oil and water.
(b) After mixing the oil and water.

When oil and water are mixed together, there is a brief moment when there will be a uniform mixture of oil and water, with drops of oil equally dispersed in the water.

Note that we are not talking here about dissolving oil in water (and creating a solution) – that is impossible, since oil is not soluble in water. We are talking about the even dispersion of oil droplets in the water. A mixture of oil and water is called an **emulsion**. When the mixing ceases, the oil will once again float to the top of the water.

To maintain the situation with the oil and water remaining uniformly mixed, we use a substance called an **emulsifier**. An emulsifier stabilizes the emulsion – the mixture of oil dispersed in water or water in oil – so that the oil and water remain 'mixed' for a long time.

There are two kinds of emulsions:

- when there is more water than oil, the oil is dispersed within the water;
- when there is more oil than water, the water is dispersed within the oil.

When the amount of water in the emulsion is relatively large, the end product is a liquid, and is called a **liquid emulsion**. If the end-product of the emulsion is in a semi-solid state, the product is a **cream**.

Creams are emulsions that appear in semi-solid form, with varying degrees of viscosity. Both liquid emulsions and creams are based on a combination of a fatty base with water. The fatty content of these preparations provide moisture to the skin.

In fact, Chapter 4, on moisturizers, deals mainly with such preparations: liquid emulsions, creams and ointments.

Liquid emulsions, creams and ointments are themselves used as bases (vehicles) in dermatological preparations.

Types of cream

There are many types of cream in cosmetics, each used for its specific purpose, and advertised under different names. Here, we shall review the main groups of creams:

- vanishing creams
- night creams
- cleansing creams
- moisturizing creams
- foundation creams
- cold creams
- eye creams

Vanishing creams
These are creams with a relatively high water content. Because of their 'watery' nature, they are easy to wash off. The water in the cream has a cooling effect. Since they do have some oil content, vanishing creams nevertheless have some moisturizing effect on the skin. However, they do not

have a significant occlusive effect (compared, for example, with ointments, which have a much higher oil content). Since vanishing creams are easier to apply, and to wash and wipe off the skin, they are usually used as day-time creams.

Usually other substances, such as sunscreens or various medications (e.g. antibiotics) or some other active ingredient (such as retinoic acid), are added to these creams.

The advantage of using a vanishing cream is, that once it has been applied to the skin, it is almost transparent, and the thin film of cream on the skin sur-face is hardly noticeable.

Various substances are promoted as vanishing creams to emphasize the fact that they are transparent, and invisible once they have been applied.

Night creams

Night creams, because of their higher oil content, are greasier and more occlu-sive than vanishing creams (but less oily and less occlusive than ointments). They are therefore used as moisturizers, and are intended for use on dry skin. They have no cooling effect.

Night creams are also known as 'nourishing' creams, since they are sup-posed to contain various substances that penetrate the skin. To enable these substances to penetrate better, the cream should remain on the skin for several hours. Hence 'nourishing' creams are applied at night, before going to bed. Because they are greasy, they tend to be more enduring, and do not drip off the skin. The 'nutritional' components of these creams com-prise various active ingredients that are supposed to have a beneficial effect on the skin once they have penetrated into the deeper skin layers. The topic of 'skin nutrition' and the effects of various cosmetic substances on the skin are dealt with in Chapter 15 on active ingredients in cosmetic prepara-tions.

Cleansing creams

These creams are discussed in Chapter 5 on skin cleansing.

Moisturizing creams

These creams, designed to increase the skin moisture content, are based on occlusives (which produce an impermeable barrier on the skin surface) and on humectants (which absorb water). This topic is dealt with in detail in Chapter 4 on skin moisture and moisturizers.

Foundation creams

Foundation creams are basically moisturizing creams. They usually contain colouring agents as well. Many of them also contain a sunscreen. As well as keeping the skin moist and protecting it from the sun, foundation creams pro-vide a smooth, even colour to the face, and are used to conceal skin blemishes. These creams are available in a range of shades, so that every woman can find the appropriate colour for her skin.

Cold creams

These are creams that have a cooling effect. The cooling occurs because these creams are 'pseudo-emulsions', rather than true emulsions: a cold cream is a simple mixture of oil and water. It does not contain an emulsifier, and so is not a stable product. Hence, when applied to the skin, the water separates from the oily component, and quickly evaporates from the skin, thus creating a cooling effect (hence the name 'cold cream').

The original cold cream was developed about 2000 years ago. In its original form, it contained olive oil, water, beeswax and rose petals, creating its characteristic aroma.

The oily component provides a cleansing effect as the cream is wiped off the skin, since the oil removes the natural oily layer of the skin surface, in which the grime particles are embedded. Cold cream can serve as a moisturizer as well because of its oily component.

Over the years, many variations on the cold cream have been developed, but the original basic composition of oil, water and wax still exists. Cosmetics companies still produce cold creams, some of which are marketed as moisturizing preparations, while with others the emphasis is on their cleansing properties, and they are marketed as cleansing preparations.

Eye creams

Preparations that are meant to be applied to the delicate skin around the eyes are mainly hypoallergenic preparations. This means that they will not contain components such as certain perfumes and/or certain preservatives that are known from past experience to have a higher than average risk of causing skin irritation and allergies. Nevertheless, there is no doubt that even eye creams may result in allergic reactions in some people.

Combining a powder with water: suspensions

As is well known, salt and sugar dissolve in water. The salt or sugar molecules are disseminated uniformly throughout the water, and the end product is called a **solution** – characterized by its clear, uniform appearance.

The substance in which the solid is dissolved (the solvent) can be water, but other substances can also function as solvents, for example alcohol (as already mentioned, a solution in alcohol is called a **tincture**). However, not all substances are soluble in water. If a water-insoluble substance, such as talc, is mixed with water, the particles of talc are large, and do not dissolve in the water. In that case, the liquid that is obtained will not appear clear and uniform.

By combining an insoluble powder with water, we obtain a **suspension**. A suspension has a cooling effect on the skin, because of the evaporation of the water. Once the water has evaporated, a layer of powder remains on the skin. It is important to shake a suspension well before applying it to the skin, so as to spread the particles of powder evenly throughout the liquid.

Combining a powder with a fatty base: pastes

A **paste** is the result of combining a powder with a fatty base. The fatty base is usually petrolatum (petroleum jelly). The powder usually comprises 20–50% of the preparation. A paste is less greasy than regular ointment, but it still has occlusive and protective properties because of its fatty content.

Because a paste contains powder, it has the ability (which an ointment lacks) of absorbing liquids to a certain extent. Under some circumstances, this gives pastes certain advantages over ointments: the main use of pastes is for protecting babies' skin from urine and stool in the diaper area. It is the contact between the infant's excretions and the skin that causes the inflammation known as **diaper rash**.

A paste may be 'hard' or 'soft'. The softer a paste, the more fatty component and the less powder it contains, and the better its skin-protective properties. The harder a paste, the more powder and the less fat it contains, and the greater its absorbent qualities. In general, pastes are not used for cosmetic purposes, but rather for dermatological uses. As stated above, the combination of their protective function together with their absorbent properties makes pastes eminently suitable for treating diaper rash in babies.

There are preparations for the treatment of diaper rash that are not pastes. Some are fatty preparations that contain substances such as allantoin or Peru balsam, which are reputed to have a 'soothing' effect.

Note: It is important to emphasize that preparations designed for use for diaper rash are only meant for simple, mild skin inflammation. If the inflammation is severe, or if there is no improvement within a reasonable time, there may be an associated bacterial or fungal infection, and in this case, the infant should be examined by a doctor.

Other combinations

Lotions

While the commonly understood meaning of the term 'lotion' covers all the liquid preparations – solutions, suspensions and emulsions – in dermatology, a lotion is sometimes regarded as a unique combination of a powder and a solution, with glycerine (glycerol) added to obtained the desired texture.

A typical and well-known example of a lotion is **calamine lotion**, widely used to treat itching. It is mainly made up of calamine (zinc oxide with a small amount of iron oxide), together with a little glycerine. As mentioned above, the glycerine contributes the appropriate texture, and moisturizes the skin to a certain degree.

A combination of a powder, water and oil

Certain liquid preparations may contain all three of these components. In this case, adding oil to the preparation helps to prevent dryness of the skin. By the same token, there are watery pastes that, in addition to the fatty and powder components, also contain water.

Note: The above definitions are the accepted medical–scientific ones. However, certain cosmetic preparations do not adhere strictly to those definitions – for example certain products may be marketed as emulsions, or 'facial cleansing emulsions', when, in fact, in terms of their composition, they are actually lotions or solutions.

Preservatives

A cosmetic or medical skin product may contain various microorganisms (bacteria or fungi) that come from the raw materials used in its manufacture, from the equipment used, from the packaging, or from exposure to the workers in the factory.

As long as the level of microorganisms is within the required standards set by the relevant authorities, there should be no complications. However, with time, these microorganisms can continue to multiply within the cosmetic preparation, which could affect the properties of the preparation and may have a deleterious effect on the skin.

The use of preservatives is a 'necessary evil'. It is better to add a preservative to a cosmetic preparation, as required by the relevant standard, than to use a defective or mouldy preparation that may contain bacteria or fungi. Bacteria tend to replicate within the watery phase of cosmetic preparations, so in products with a high water content there is a higher risk of bacterial or fungal contamination.

How can contaminated products be recognized?

A substance infected by bacteria develops an unpleasant smell. Generally, it loses its uniform texture, and there is a definite separation into its two phases: watery and oily. There may be various discoloured areas on the surface of the product – these discoloured patches are, in fact, colonies of bacteria or mould.

To prevent this from happening, cosmetics manufacturers add preservatives to prevent the growth of bacteria or fungi in their preparations.

More details about preservatives

The shelf life of a cosmetic or medical product depends on the conditions under which it is stored. The more appropriate the storage conditions, the more stable the product. After leaving the manufacturer, it should not be exposed to sunlight or high temperatures; most cosmetic and medical products should be stored in a cool, dark, dry place. Only products displaying an expiry date should be used.

It is important to avoid leaving bits of paper or cotton-wool inside the container after using the product, since these are the main sources of bacterial contamination.

Cosmetic or medical preparations should not be transferred to empty jars. Similarly, remnants of an older product should not be mixed with a fresh product of the same type, since this may lead to contamination of the latter.

A cosmetic product whose colour texture or smell has changed should not be used.

Common preservatives used in cosmetics

These preservatives, which may be listed on the package, include:

- Benzoic acid
- Benzyl alcohol
- Formaldehyde
- Imidazolidinyl urea
- Parabens
- Quaternium 15

Summary

- The base of any cosmetic or medical product for use on the skin is either a fatty base, water, powder, or various combinations thereof.
- By using these bases or various combinations of them, different types of cosmetic and medical products are produced: powders, aqueous solutions, ointments, creams, emulsions, suspensions, pastes and lotions.
- An active ingredient and other supplementary substances (where necessary) are added to the base, to produce the final product.

Addendum: gels

Similar to the bases discussed earlier, a **gel** may also function as a base for various cosmetic and medical skin preparations. A gel is a semi-solid, non-greasy, colourless, transparent substance. Gels tend to evaporate when in contact with warm skin, or when rubbed onto the skin.

Composition of gels

In its basic form, a gel is a solution, where the solvent may be water, acetone, alcohol or propylene glycol. Another type of gel is one whose basic state is that of a liquid emulsion: in other words, an oil–water combination. However, whether we are speaking of a gel that is basically a solution or one that is basically a liquid emulsion, there is an additional modification: in gels, the original preparation undergoes a process of thickening by the addition of various substances, resulting in a more viscous and less watery product – the extent depending on the desired degree of viscosity. The higher level of viscosity enables a gel preparation to adhere better and to 'stick' to the skin, and to stay longer on the skin surface, compared with liquid preparations.

When is a gel preferable to a cream?

Since creams do not contain thickeners, they need to contain a higher amount of fatty base in order to achieve the same degree of viscosity and 'stickiness' as a gel. Hence, if we wanted a preparation to contain as little fatty components as possible, yet be viscous, we would prefer a gel over a cream. Therefore gels are usually designed for use on oily skin, where we do not want to use an oily substance but prefer a more watery preparation.

4

Skin moisture and moisturizers

Contents   Skin moisture: overview • What causes dry skin? • Significance of skin moisture: characteristics of dry skin • What are the beneficial effects of moisturizers? • Natural factors that prevent skin dryness • Wetting the skin • Moisturizers: occlusives and humectants • How to select a moisturizer • Guidelines for use of moisturizers • What is the difference between moisturizers for the face and those for the rest of the body? • Moisturizers for the hands • Summary

Skin moisture: overview

The water content in the viable skin (dermis and epidermis) is approximately 80%. The outer skin layer, the keratinous layer, is made of dead skin cells with a lower water content, approximately 10–30%.

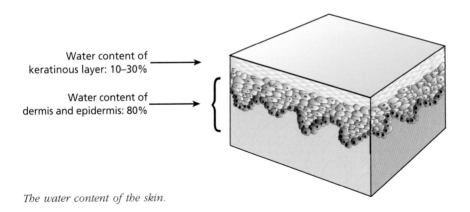

Water content of keratinous layer: 10–30%

Water content of dermis and epidermis: 80%

The water content of the skin.

This water content allows the keratinous layer a certain amount of suppleness. When the water content of the skin is normal, the skin appears soft, smooth, supple and glowing. The skin is slightly swollen, so there is a certain flattening of the skin surface, with fading of fine wrinkles.

In normal skin, there is a continuous movement of water from the deep layers of the skin to the superficial layers. Eventually, the water evaporates from the surface.

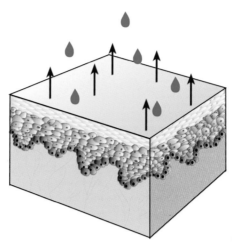

Evaporation of water from the skin surface.

What causes dry skin?

Dry skin is relatively common: most people will experience skin dryness, to some extent, from time to time. Dry skin can result from external causes as well as from changes in the skin's ability to retain its moisture.

External causes

The major external causes are exposure to a dry environment and wind.

Note that artificial indoor heating lowers the relative humidity even further. Therefore the skin tends to be dryer in the winter. Staying for prolonged periods in an air-conditioned room, with cold, dry air being blown into the room, can cause the skin to become dry as well.

Other external influences on the dryness of the skin include the following:

- **Washing:** frequent washing repeatedly removes the oily layer that protects the skin. Certain types of soaps have a particularly drying effect.
- **Exposure to certain substances:** various occupations are characterized by exposure to substances that remove the natural oily layer from the skin surface, such as those occupations involving frequent exposure to detergents or solvents. Similarly, certain medical treatments (such as some for acne) cause drying of the skin.

The skin's ability to retain moisture

Ageing is associated with physiological processes whereby the skin loses its ability to retain moisture. Furthermore, there are diseases in which the skin does not retain body water normally, and significant amounts of water are lost through the skin. This occurs, for example, in **atopic dermatitis** and in certain other skin disorders resulting from dietary deficiencies.

Significance of skin moisture: characteristics of dry skin

Skin with a low water content appears dry, fissured and rough. It has a delicate layer of scales on its surface. Fine lines are more apparent. The individual perceives a feeling of dryness, which may be accompanied by itching.

Dry skin is more prone to skin infections, both bacterial and fungal. The common dermatological term for extremely dry skin is **xerosis**.

Dry skin.

Dry skin

Dry skin loses its suppleness in proportion to the decrease in its water content. Skin with a normal moisture content will slough off dead cells naturally. In dry skin, the superficial layers do not peel off easily, and remain attached. The accumulated keratinous cells are manifested as scales on the dry skin.

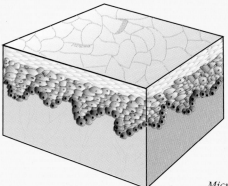

Microscopic structure of dry skin.

In addition, extremely dry skin, which is tough and less pliable, tends to fissure. These fissures damage the integrity and continuity of the skin, and interfere with its function as a protective layer. Subsequently, there is increased water loss, and the skin becomes dryer, more fissures appear, and the process is aggravated.

What are the beneficial effects of moisturizers?

In stark contrast to advertisements concerning the 'anti-ageing', 'age-reversing' qualities of certain moisturizing products, it has never been proven that moisturizers prevent the ageing process caused by advanced age or sun exposure. However, use of moisturizers may benefit the skin in numerous ways:

- **Preventing damage caused by dryness**: This has been described previously.
- **Protection**: The thin oily layer on the skin surface can protect it from exposure to environmental factors such as soot particles, dirt and dust.
- **Temporary aesthetic improvement**: As previously stated, when the skin is well moisturized, it appears *temporarily* smoother and more refreshed. Since it is slightly swollen, there is flattening and virtual obliteration of fine wrinkles. The pores also appear somewhat smaller, since the skin surrounding them is slightly swollen. This temporary improvement is exploited by advertisers, in marketing various moisturizing products, claiming an 'anti-ageing' effect.

Nevertheless, protection from environmental factors and damage caused by dryness is significant in determining skin texture. It prevents a deterioration in the appearance and quality of facial skin.

Note: Not everyone requires moisturizers, and individuals with oily skin usually have no use for them. However, during exposure to dry environmental conditions, such as dry air and cold wind, they may be needed. Older people, whose skin is usually dryer, may require such products more frequently.

Natural factors that prevent skin dryness

The skin is protected naturally from dryness by an occlusive oily layer and by a natural moisturizing factor.

An occlusive, oily layer on the skin – the lipid film

The lipid film decreases water evaporation. It serves as an occlusive layer above the keratin layer. This layer is a combination of oily products on the skin surface, and includes mainly:

- the sebum secreted by the sebaceous glands;
- various lipid degradation products that are formed during the process of skin maturation: when the epidermal cells traverse upwards, chemical changes occur in them; eventually, cell death occurs, and various degradation products, partly lipid, are formed.

Natural moisturizing factor (NMF)

This is a combination of several compounds created in the skin and comprising approximately 20–25% of the keratinous layer. These compounds retain the water content of the keratinous layer.

Natural moisturizing factor (NMF)

Among the compounds that compose the NMF are:

- urea
- lactic acid
- glycolic acid
- phospholipids
- malic acid
- pyruvic acid
- salts of pyrrolidone carboxylic acid

(We mention these compounds since some may appear in various moisturizers and may be listed on the packaging.)

Wetting the skin

Wetting of the skin can be achieved in two ways:

- soaking
- repeated washing or repeated application of a damp cloth

Prolonged soaking

When the hand is soaked in water, the water penetrates the skin. If the soaking is prolonged, the water may cause damage. At first, the keratinous layer appears swollen and pale. At a later stage, maceration of the skin appears and the damage is more pronounced. An increase of the moisture to such a level causes a predisposition to infections, both bacterial and fungal, in the skin of the hands.

Repeated washing or repeated placing of a damp cloth on skin

When we allow the water that we have added (by washing or repeatedly placing a damp cloth on skin) to evaporate, a different situation arises. Here, the added water evaporates, and with it, 'pulls' water previously located in the outer layers of the skin.

Thus the quantity of water evaporated is *greater* than that which was applied. Finally, the skin's water content is smaller than it was at the beginning of the washing process. This phenomenon seems paradoxical – however, frequent washing of the skin with water does have a drying effect.

In dermatology, physicians apply this principle for drying inflamed and secreting skin areas by repeated washing, several times a day, each time for a few minutes.

Moisturizers: occlusives and humectants

Hence water is not useful for retaining sufficient skin moisture. In order to preserve skin moisture one must apply moisturizers.

There are two principal methods for preserving the moisture of the skin:

- using occlusives
- using humectants

Occlusives

These substances produce an oily layer on the skin, enriching the skin's natural lipid film, which prevents water evaporation. The keratinous layer dampens, becoming more fully saturated with water.

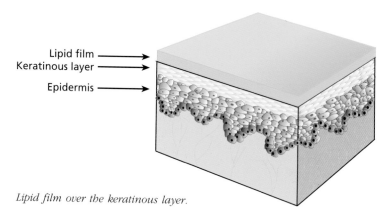

Lipid film ⟶
Keratinous layer ⟶
Epidermis ⟶

Lipid film over the keratinous layer.

These products are more effective if applied directly after washing, trapping a layer of water beneath them. Substances such as the following can be used:

- mineral-derived fatty compounds such as paraffin or petroleum jelly (the most common mineral source is crude oil, from which various oils can be derived after refining); cetomacrogol is another occlusive, mineral-derived compound that can be found in various moisturizers;
- substances derived from animal fat, such as lanolin and its derivatives (derived from sheep's wool);
- vegetable oils such as olive oil, oat oil, peanut oil and sesame seed oil, and many others.

Vegetable oils are less occlusive than animal-derived oils or mineral oil, yet allow sufficient occlusion.

Note: Oily products all function in the same way, preventing water evaporation from the superficial layers of the skin. There is no significant difference among the various fatty products derived from animals. None have any proven age-reversing abilities. Oils derived from rare animals are not superior, and their use is only an uncalled-for commercial gimmick.

Some moisturizing products contain a substance called **spermaceti**, which is produced from whales. The use of these products is prohibited in the USA. Those consumers who have reservations about the killing of whales should avoid using products containing this substance: one can read the label of contents on the product to ensure that it does not contain spermaceti.

It should be remembered that occlusive products tend to be sticky and oily, so consumers will generally refrain from using products that appear in an oilier form (such as an ointment). Therefore these products are generally combined as creams or lotions (which have a greater water content). These are easier to apply, and are preferred by most consumers. After water evaporation, the occlusive components that remain will protect the skin and fulfil their function.

Humectants

These products absorb water. This group includes a large number of substances, some of which are able to penetrate the keratinous layer, thereby increasing its water content.

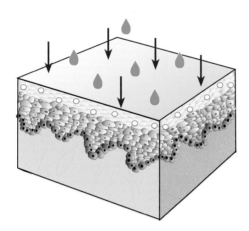

Water-absorbing substances (shown as clear circles) in the keratinous layer.

Other products from this group have large molecules that do not penetrate the keratinous layer, but form a hygroscopic (water-absorbing) layer on the skin. The effectiveness of several of these products is debatable. In a relatively arid environment, they may actually absorb water from the skin (rather than the environment), causing increased dryness. On the other hand, in a humid environment, they are clearly efficient. In conclusion, their efficacy is not as great as occlusive products in a cold, dry environment.

Therefore an efficient moisturizer, suited to cold, dry weather, should contain a combination of occlusives and humectants.

In daily usage, moisturizing cosmetics made only from water-absorbing substances are called **non-oily moisturizers**.

Humectants

The products in use are as follows:

Products composed of relatively small molecules with efficient absorbing capabilities:

- glycerine (glycerol)
- sorbitol
- propylene glycol

Macromolecules
Products composed of larger molecules that are not able to penetrate the keratinous layer form a hygroscopic, water-absorbing layer on the skin. These include:

- glycosaminoglycans (such as hyaluronic acid)
- elastin, collagen, and other proteins

Components of the natural moisturizing factor (NMF)
The humectant group includes other products with absorbing capabilities. Since the NMF was identified, it was only logical to use its components in order to increase skin moisture. These components include:

- the sodium salt of pyrollidone carboxylic acid
- urea (in 10–20% concentrations)
- lactic acid
- phospholipids

Note that lactic acid belongs to the group of alpha-hydroxy acids. These have been introduced for cosmetic and dermatological use in recent years, and are notable for their ability to increase the water content of the skin.

The liposomes found in various cosmetic products are made up of phospholipids. Products containing liposomes also have a certain ability to increase the skin's moisture level (in addition to other advantages of the liposomes).

Detailed descriptions of alpha-hydroxy acids and liposomes appear in Chapters 17 and 21 respectively.

In order to identify which moisturizers contain humectants, one can read the label of contents on the package and refer to the above list.

From a practical point of view, the various approaches to skin moisturizing are not distinctly segregated. Most moisturizers have a number of components from each group. They usually contain occlusive, oily products along with humectants. In addition, a number of the components have a combined effect: lanolin and its derivatives, for example, have occlusive as well as absorptive properties.

How to select a moisturizer

Hundreds of moisturizers are available. They may contain substances previously mentioned. They may contain occlusive products, water-absorbing products, or a combination of these. They are sold in various formulations:

- liquid emulsions
- ointments
- creams

The water content and lipid components differ in each formula type. Products rich in water are cool to the touch, and appear matte; products with a higher oil content cause a warm sensation, and the skin appears smooth and glossy.

How does one determine the preferred moisturizer?

Skin type

The foremost factor in selecting a moisturizer in skin type, determined by its lipid content.

Dry skin

Dry skin lacks sheen. The pores are hardly noticeable. These individuals usually have lighter-toned skin. In extreme cases, as previously detailed, the skin will be scaly and fissured.

Oily skin

Oily skin is glossy, especially on the forehead, nose and chin. The skin is oily to the touch. Large pores are apparent. Individuals with this type of skin tend to suffer from acne as adolescents.

Normal skin

This is somewhere between dry and oily skin. The skin is neither glossy nor oily to the touch, yet appears smooth and well-moisturized. The pores are not large.

'Combination skin'

This skin type is almost identical to the normal skin type. The T-zone, which includes the forehead, nasal bridge, nose and centre of the chin, has an increased level of sebaceous gland activity. The skin tends to be oily in these areas.

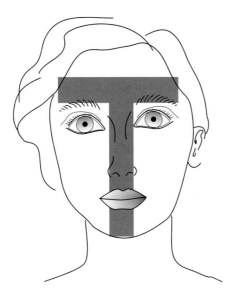

The T-zone: forehead, nasal bridge, nose and centre of the chin.

Note: Skin type must be determined on a 'clean' face. No conclusions should be drawn concerning the quality of skin when a moisturizer has recently been applied, or the skin has recently been washed with a drying soap.

Which moisturizers should be used for which types of skin?

For an **individual with dry facial skin**, using moisturizers containing only humectants will not be enough. Oily moisturizers containing occlusive components are required. If the skin is fairly 'normal' and not dry, one should use a preparation that has both occlusives and humectants (water-absorbing products).

An **individual with oily skin or a tendency towards oily skin** does not need moisturizers (except at those times when the face becomes drier, for example following exposure to a cold wind). Similarly, one should avoid applying moisturizers on **acne-affected skin**.

For skin that is **normal or near-normal**, one should use a moisturizing preparation that incorporates less of the oily, occlusive substances. In this case, preparations containing humectants are recommended.

If the skin type is **combined and it is oilier in the T-zone of the face**, one should avoid applying moisturizing preparations in the T-zone. On the rest of the face, one should use non-oily products (containing humectants).

Note: It should be remembered that the skin tends to dry with age. An individual who did not require moisturizers in the past may require them later in life. Changes in the environment, or a shift to an arid environment, will require moisturizers as well. Seasonal changes may cause one to feel a need for moisturizing products, such as in winter.

In addition to the skin type, there are other variables that may influence the choice of a moisturizer:

- **Consistency**: The product's texture and consistency is a significant factor. Certainly a product that is not pleasant to the touch, such as one that feels sticky or oily, should not be selected. The flood of products on the market enables the consumer to select a moisturizer perfectly suited to one's aesthetic needs.
- **Additives**: Fragrances and preservatives may irritate and sensitize. For some individuals, it is necessary to avoid using products containing these components, which may cause skin irritation, or are not necessarily required. Cosmetics companies are currently manufacturing hypoallergenic products, which may contain fewer potentially allergenic compounds. These may be preferred for sensitized individuals. However, even cosmetic products labeled as 'hypoallergenic' may contain various preservatives and fragrances as well, with the potential to induce allergic reactions.

  Products marketed as eye creams should be formulated to minimize irritation and redness of the eyes. Obviously, products that may irritate are not recommended for use on the skin in general, and on the skin surrounding the eye in particular.
- **Sunscreens**: There is no justification for using a moisturizer containing sunscreens if it is planned for evening or night use. However, it may be recommended to use a moisturizing lotion that contains an efficient sunscreen, if applied in areas exposed to the sun during daytime.
- **'Exotic' ingredients**: Exotic ingredients such as allantoin, gelatin, vitamins, proteins and royal bee jelly are not superior to conventional compounds in retaining skin moisture. There is no scientific evidence that they have additional benefits, such as age-reversing qualities.

Various preparations, including exotic ingredients in cosmetic products, are detailed in Chapter 15 on active ingredients in cosmetic preparations.

Guidelines for use of moisturizers

As a rule, individuals with dry skin should avoid frequent washing of the face with soap; they should also avoid exposure to harsh environmental factors such as cold wind and dry weather.

The application of moisturizers after skin cleansing may be recommended. The product should be applied after washing, when the skin is still slightly damp. Application should be gentle. Excess scrubbing is unnecessary, and may irritate.

The frequency of application should be determined according to skin type. Dry skin will require more frequent application of moisturizers. Extremely dry skin requires numerous daily applications, depending on the product used.

The moisturizer should be applied to the face and neck. If the T-zone (forehead, nasal bridge, nose and chin) is oily, one should avoid moisturizing this area unnecessarily.

Note: Moisturizers that contain relatively large amounts of water (i.e. liquid emulsions or creams) should not be applied just before exposure to cold weather. In this case, the wet skin is exposed to the drying effect of the cold wind. As water on the skin's surface evaporates, it has a cooling effect. Cold, dry conditions may harm facial skin. One should consider the following:

- Apply the moisturizer 20–30 minutes prior to exposure to a cold, dry or windy environment.
- Under these conditions, oily moisturizers may be preferable.

What is the difference between moisturizers for the face and those for the rest of the body?

In principle, there is no significant difference between moisturizers designed for the face and those for the rest of the body. Any moisturizer that increases the moisture of the face will also be effective in increasing the moisture elsewhere. Nevertheless, since applying moisturizer to the body involves much larger areas, manufacturers generally make body moisturizers in the form of liquid emulsions (rather than creams or ointments), to make them easier to apply. Clearly, this is not a rigid rule. There are some facial moisturizers that appear in a liquid form, and there are many body moisturizers in the form of creams or ointments.

Most people will take more care to apply moisturizer to the face and neck than elsewhere, because of the aesthetic importance of the skin in these regions, and also because those areas are more exposed to the vagaries of the environment, such as sun and wind.

Some body moisturizers are meant to be used in the bath or shower, for people with particularly dry skin. The advantage is that while bathing, a layer of water is trapped between the skin and the moisturizer, which further increases the moisture content of the skin. Each preparation comes with detailed instructions as to how much to add to the bathwater, for both infants and adults.

Moisturizers for the hands

Moisturizers designed for the hands are based on the same principles as other moisturizers. They contain occlusives or humectants, or a combination of both. However, there is another aspect to hand moisturizers: the skin of the hands is subjected to repeated washing with soap and water. Therefore moisturizers for the hands contain oils that may be water-resistant, which create an impermeable, occlusive layer on the skin that does not wash off easily.

Furthermore, hand moisturizers often contain an additional ingredient: **oil-based silicone**. This substance is water-repellent. Owing to the presence of this water-repellent silicone layer, the natural lipid film on the skin is not washed away, and the skin remains moist.

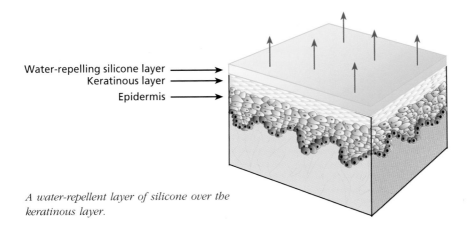

Water-repelling silicone layer ⟶
Keratinous layer ⟶
Epidermis ⟶

A water-repellent layer of silicone over the keratinous layer.

These products may be effective in protecting the skin of the hands, which is repeatedly subject to washing with soap and water. For people engaged in manual work involving exposing their hands to various harsh substances, silicone-containing moisturizers may provide a layer protecting the skin from toxic substances, allergens (substances producing allergic reactions) and irritants. The degree of moisture achievable with these substances is, in general, less than that achieved by using occlusive or water-absorbent substances. However, as stated earlier, the presence of a water-repellent layer on the skin may be a possible advantage.

Summary

- Moisturizers are made up of occlusive substances, water-absorbent substances (humectants), or combinations of the two.
- The use of a moisturizer must be adjusted to the type of skin.
- For dry skin, one needs an oily moisturizer that contains a relatively higher concentration of occlusive compounds.
- For normal or near-normal skin, it is advisable to use a moisturizer that combines an occlusive substance with a water-absorbent substance. The skin type also determines the frequency of application of a moisturizer. The drier the skin, the more often it should be used.
- Moisturizers should be applied gently, after cleaning the skin and washing it with water.

5
Skin cleansing

Contents   Skin cleansing: overview • How does soap work? Soap and its mode of action • Disadvantages of regular soap • What is pH? • Synthetic soaps ('soapless soap') • What does soap contain other than the active ingredient? • 'Mild'/hypoallergenic soaps • Soaps for use in acne • Washing the face

Skin cleansing: overview

Cleansing the skin is basic to maintaining its health, and contributes to the aesthetic appearance of the skin.

What is the dirt that has to be removed?
It is made up of:

- dust
- soot (from the air)
- sweat
- breakdown products of sebum
- residues of cosmetics and make-up that were applied onto the skin
- other substances carried in the air, which vary depending on the geographical location and the environment

All the above substances stick to the thin, oily layer on the surface of the skin. Since the dirt is embedded in the oily layer, obviously washing with water is not sufficient to cleanse the skin. Water is repelled by the oil, and therefore is not able to remove the oily layer of the skin surface containing the dirt particles. As anyone who has ever tried to wash oil off the hands with water knows, water alone cannot remove oil or fat. To effectively remove the fine oily layer on the skin surface, in which the dirt is embedded, one obviously has to use soap.

How does soap work? Soap and its mode of action

The active ingredients in soap are salts of various fatty acids.

> **Fatty acids commonly used in soaps**
>
> Stearic acid
> Palmitic acid
> Oleic acid
> Myristic acid
> Lauric acid

In terms of its basic chemical composition, regular, classic soap, known as **hard soap** or **toilet soap**, comprises the sodium salts of fatty acids. These fatty acids are derived from either animal or vegetable sources.

Because of soap's particular molecular structure, the soap particles 'coat' the fat droplets in which the dirt is embedded, and allow them to be washed off the skin with water. These soap structures that coat the fat (and dirt) particles, and allow them to be removed from the skin, are called **micelles**. The soap molecules arrange themselves in the form of micelles because of the electric charge they carry. The soap micelles surround the fat droplet, and thus enable its removal from the skin.

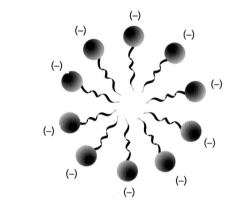

A soap micelle.

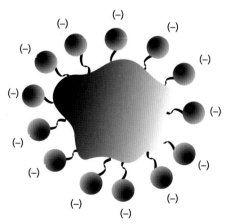

A micelle coating a fat droplet.

Disadvantages of regular soap

Normal tap water contains calcium and magnesium. As a result, when ordinary soap is used, calcium and magnesium salts of fatty acids are formed. These are 'sticky' salts that are not readily soluble. The salts are left on the skin surface, and may lead to skin irritation.

Another reason regular soap may cause skin irritation is that it has a high pH. The pH of regular soap lies between 9 and 10 (and sometimes higher than 10) – much higher than the normal skin pH (which is between 4 and 6.5). Consequently, the effect of regular soap coming in contact with the skin is to raise the skin's pH. (See below for an explanation of the concept of pH.)

It is true, however, that healthy skin has mechanisms for adjusting its pH, so that a short time after it has been exposed to regular soap, its level of acidity returns to normal. (Various research studies have shown that the pH returns to normal any time from half an hour to two hours after soap has been used.) Nevertheless, in some people, abrupt changes in pH, particularly increases in pH, can cause significant skin irritation. Therefore the current trend in the cosmetics industry is to adapt the pH of cleansing agents and other cosmetic preparations to that of normal skin.

> ### Skin acidity protects against infections
>
> The acidity of the skin is a protective mechanism of the body against bacterial and fungal infections. The natural pH of the skin acts as a protective acid mantle.

What is pH?

pH is a numerical value that expresses the acidity of a solution. The acidity of a solution is determined by the concentration of hydrogen ions in it. pH values range from 0 to 14. The actual value of the pH of a solution is derived from a logarithmic calculation based on the concentration of hydrogen ions in the solution.

- a very strong **acid** (such as hydrochloric acid), has a high concentration of hydrogen ions, and a pH close to 0;
- a very strong **base**, or **alkali** (such as sodium hydroxide), has a low concentration of hydrogen ions, and a pH close to 14;
- the pH of pure water, which is **neutral**, is 7;
- the pH of blood is 7.4;
- the pH of milk varies from 6 to 7;

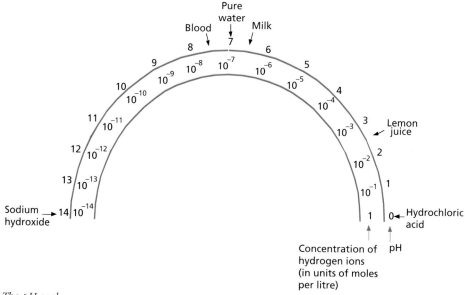

The pH scale.

- the pH of lemon juice is between 2 and 3;
- the normal skin pH ranges from 4 to 6.5.

Synthetic soaps ('soapless soap')

The disadvantages of regular soap created the need for new soaps. As early as the 1940s, cosmetics companies started manufacturing synthetic soaps, largely derived from by-products of crude oil refining.

Surfactants, or **surface-active agents**, are water-soluble compounds that make up the major component of soaps and shampoos. The surface-active agents in newer soaps act in exactly the same way as was described for regular soap:

- Because of their electric charge, they form micelles.
- Small particles of oil are trapped inside the micelles.
- In that way, the oil and particles of dirt embedded within it can be washed off with water.

All the other cleansing agents made of surface-active agents are called:

- artificial soaps, or
- soapless soaps, or
- non-soaps, or
- synthetic soaps,

and they may be in the form of solids or liquids.

Surfactants

There are four groups of surfactants:

- anionics
- cationics
- non-ionics
- amphoterics

The nature of each group is determined by its chemical charge – as can be seen in the illustration below. Each surfactant group has different chemical properties that affect the way it cleans.

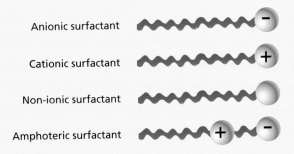

The regular soaps discussed above are, in terms of their chemical structure, sodium salts of fatty acids. They belong to the anionic surfactant group.

Clarification regarding the term 'detergent'

Some people include any cleaning agent under this definition. However, the term 'synthetic detergent' usually refers to a 'soapless soap'. In general, manufacturers avoid using the term 'detergent' in relation to skin cleansing agents or shampoos; they prefer to use the terms 'soapless soap', or 'surfactant'. This is because the average person tends to associate the word 'detergent' with those strong detergents used for cleaning dishes, etc. In fact, all detergents accomplish their cleaning action by the same principle described in this chapter.

Advantages of synthetic soaps

Synthetic soaps usually cause less skin irritation than regular soap does. The pH of synthetic soaps can be adjusted to that of the normal skin by the addition of substances such as lactic acid of citric acid.

What does soap contain other than the active ingredient?

As already stated, the active ingredients in all cleansing agents and soaps are surface-active agents. Nevertheless, apart from surfactants, soaps contain other ingredients:

- moisturizers
- preservatives
- colouring agents
- fragrances and perfumes
- antibacterial substances
- substances that alter the pH
- other ingredients

Moisturizers

All soaps tend to remove the oily layer on the skin surface. However, it is not only the oil containing the dirt particles that is removed – the soap also removes the natural oily layer on the skin, which is important for skin protection. Hence the use of soap, with the consequent removal of the natural oily layer, dries the skin. Loss of the oily protective layer also increases the likelihood of irritation.

For this reason, soaps contain moisturizing agents, such as lanolin, glycerine and various vegetable fats. These substances leave a thin protective layer on the skin, to counteract the drying effect of the soap. However, both the action of the soap itself (in removing oily substances) and the rinsing with water remove soap moisturizers from the skin. Thus significant amounts of moisturizers will not be left on the skin surface following the use of soap. Therefore anyone who has a tendency to dry skin should apply moisturizing agents in the form of creams or ointments, and not rely on the use of soaps containing moisturizers.

Moisturizing agents are dealt with in Chapter 4.

Soaps meant for use on oily skin

These soaps contain minimal amounts, if any, of moisturizing agents. In addition, they contain surfactants that are particularly effective in removing the oily layer from the skin. In general, the use of moisturizing agents should be tailored to the type of skin: someone with dry skin needs a soap that contains moisturizing agents. On the other hand, there is no need (and indeed it is unwise) for someone with oily skin, or someone with acne, to use moisturizing soap.

Transparent soaps

These represent another type of soap containing moisturizers. These soaps usually contain a higher than usual concentration of glycerine, or various sugars. The high glycerine content gives the soap its transparent appearance.

Some dermatologists maintain that glycerine tends to absorb water out of the skin, and thereby these soaps may have a drying effect in certain cases. For this reason, some transparent soaps contain additional moisturizing agents; hence each transparent soap can be tailored specifically for dry, normal or oily skin. In general, transparent soaps are considered to be relatively mild.

Preservatives and colouring agents

These substances are dealt with in detail in Chapter 3 on the preparation of medical and cosmetic products

Fragrances and perfumes

As is common practice in most cosmetic preparations, scents of various types are usually added to soaps, to hide the odours of the raw ingredients of the soap. Sometimes these substances can cause allergic reactions.

Antibacterial substances

'Antibacterial soaps' usually contain triclocarban and triclosan. Residues of these substances remain on the skin surface after washing, and inhibit the growth of bacteria.

Soaps that contain antibacterial substances are used mainly to prevent unpleasant body odours. They are also used for several types of superficial skin infections (such as folliculitis – infection of the hair follicles – or acne), as well as following exposure to dirt or any potential source of contamination.

Apocrine glands and unpleasant body odours

These result from the breakdown of organic substances present in the secretions of certain types of sweat glands, called **apocrine glands**, found in the armpits and groin. These substances are broken down by bacteria. Hence using antibacterial soaps that inhibit the growth of bacteria prevents, to a certain extent, the formation of unpleasant body odour.

The antibacterial effect of these soaps depends on how often they are used during the day. Since there are no apocrine sweat glands on the face, and if the purpose of these soaps is to prevent body odour, their use should be confined to washing the body.

Unpleasant body odour derived from the apocrine glands in the armpits and groin develops after puberty. Therefore there is no justification using these soaps in children for this purpose.

There are other soaps with antibacterial properties:

- Some soaps contain benzoyl peroxide: this substance is an antimicrobial agent, and is used in the treatment of acne. See the section later in this chapter on soaps used in the treatment of acne.
- Soaps containing a high concentration of lactic acid have a pH of about 3.5. These soaps are said to have some antibacterial action.
- Soaps containing povidone iodine – an iodine-based antibacterial compound – have marked antibacterial properties, but can cause skin irritation. They should therefore be used only after consulting a physician, who will advise whether there is a medical problem that justifies their use. Gynaecologists sometimes recommend some of these soaps for vaginal douching.

Substances that alter skin pH

Substances that alter skin pH are usually acids, such as lactic or citric acid. The aim is generally to adjust the pH of the substance to the normal pH of healthy skin (the normal value is between 4 and 6.5). Certain soaps are designed to deliberately lower the skin pH, since lowering the skin pH is supposed to produce some antibacterial effect.

Other ingredients

Certain soaps contain other ingredients, such as vitamins, various medical preparations and a variety of exotic 'natural' ingredients (usually derived from fruits, other plants, etc.). In most cases, these additives are of no documented medical value. Soap is in contact with the skin for a brief period only, and, in any case, if the soap 'performs' as it is supposed to, these substances would be quickly washed off the skin.

The effect of any additive on the skin must be considered. If a certain ingredient really does benefit the skin, it would be preferable to use some other cosmetic preparation (such as a cream or an emulsion) containing the required ingredient. That way, by applying the preparation to the skin, the substance in it will be in contact with the skin for a longer period, and may truly have some beneficial effect on the skin.

'Mild'/hypoallergenic soaps

These are soaps from which certain ingredients, such as fragrances and colouring agents, have been removed. The substances excluded from the soap are those that, statistically, have a higher chance of causing skin irritation or allergic reactions. Another feature of these soaps is that they may contain substances from the betaine group, which are amphoteric surfactants. These are known to be relatively 'mild', and do not tend to cause stinging of the skin or eyes.

Nevertheless, even 'mild' and hypoallergenic soaps can cause skin irritation and allergic reactions – although the likelihood of this happening is theoretically less than with regular soaps.

Hypoallergenic soaps are designed for use by people with delicate skin and for infants.

Soaps for use in acne

As noted above, some of the soaps intended for use in acne contain antibacterial substances such as benzoyl peroxide. Benzoyl peroxide is a strong oxidizing agent that penetrates the hair follicle and acts on the bacteria that are involved in the development of acne.

The other soaps intended for use in acne are mainly those designed for use on oily skin, which have very potent cleansing properties. Reducing the oiliness of the skin may help in the treatment of acne. Note, however, that most of the medical preparations used nowadays in the treatment of acne dry out the skin, and one must take care not to end up with extremely dry skin because of the excessive use of soaps that tend to dry the skin, together with medical preparations that are applied to the skin and that also dry out the skin.

Washing the face

- A mild soap, suited to the skin type, should be used. For dry skin, soap with moisturizer should be used.
- Excessive scrubbing of the face while washing is unnecessary.
- When drying the face, vigorous rubbing, which may irritate the skin, should be avoided. The face can be wiped by gently dabbing with a soft towel.
- Lukewarm water – not too hot and not too cold – should be used.

6

Creams and liquid emulsions for facial cleansing

Contents Overview • What possible advantages are there in creams and liquid emulsions for facial cleansing? • Cleansing cream should not be used as moisturizing cream • Abrasive cleansers • Summary

Note: This chapter should be read after Chapter 5 on skin cleansing.

Overview

Creams and liquid emulsions for cleansing the face are basically mixtures of oil and water. The difference between a cream and a liquid emulsion is in their degree of viscosity. When the preparation is thin and fluid, we speak of a **liquid emulsion**; if the preparation contains more fatty components, so that it is semi-solid, we speak of a **cream**. Both creams and liquid emulsions intended for facial cleansing are composed of oils, water and cleansing substances (usually the same substances as are found in the 'mild' soaps), with the proportions between the various components differing from product to product.

Facial cleansing creams and emulsions are composed (among other ingredients) of soap, through which the cleansing effect occurs. However, they also contain oil and water. Therefore, while soap disperses the oil (and the dirt particles embedded in it) found in the fatty layer of the skin into the tap water being added in rinsing off the mixture of soap and oil, the cleansing creams and emulsions disperse the oil particles from the skin **within themselves**. These preparations should be applied to the skin with the fingertips, and left on the skin briefly. When they are removed from the skin with a tissue or a wet facecloth, or by rinsing off with water (preferred!), the fatty layer with the dissolved dirt is removed with them.

As with other cosmetic preparations, the cosmetics industry adds various ancillary substances to cleansing creams and emulsions; **emulsifiers** to stabilize the product, **antiseptics** (to act against bacteria), various solvents and moisturizers.

What possible advantages are there in creams and liquid emulsions for facial cleansing?

Make-up preparations, especially those based on heavy oils, are removed from the skin more easily using cleansing creams or emulsions, which have a relatively high fat content compared with normal soap. Cleansing creams and emulsions dissolve the fatty substances (which contain the make-up pigments) within themselves, making removal of make-up easier.

These substances are more effective at removing sebum from the skin than is rubbing the skin with soap and water.

Since cleansing creams and emulsions contain oils, a thin layer of oil may still remain on the skin after rinsing them off. For this reason, these preparations are generally more effective for people with dry skin (and are not usually recommended for people with oily skin or acne). Nevertheless, many cleansing creams and preparations are manufactured in a range of variations, as sub-groups of the original product, designated specifically for use with dry, normal or oily skin – depending on the customer's requirements.

Cleansing creams and emulsions are usually made of relatively delicate cleansing agents (compared with the wide variety of soaps and 'soapless soaps'). If they are rinsed off with water after use (and not just wiped off), their cleansing effect is gentler, and usually does not cause skin irritation.

Cleansing cream should not be used as moisturizing cream

Since cleansing creams and emulsions contain cleansing agents, they should be removed from the skin as soon as possible, since they are liable to cause skin irritation if left in contact with the skin for too long. Leaving a cleansing cream on the skin, as one does with a moisturizing cream, is the same as leaving soap on the skin – not a good idea! Furthermore, for this reason, it is definitely preferable to wash cleansing creams and emulsions off with water, and not merely wipe them off the skin with a paper tissue or cloth.

Abrasive cleansers

Abrasive cleansers are creams or emulsions designed for cleaning the face. In addition to the standard ingredients described above, the 'abrasive effect' is achieved by the presence of tiny, fine granules – some natural and some made of synthetic compounds. These preparations are supposed to remove the keratin layer of the skin that normally peels off. This is achieved by mechanical means, by the abrasive effect of the granules on the skin. Removing the outermost layers of keratin may help produce a uniform, smooth surface on the skin, and improve its appearance.

In spite of the fact that these preparations are effective in removing the peeling skin layers, there is no proof that they offer any additional benefit in cleaning the skin, or caring for it, compared with soaps or other facial cleansing creams or emulsions. In general, healthy, normal skin does not require such treatment. The outermost layers of skin are normally constantly peeling off, and do not need any assistance in doing so! Furthermore, several dermatologists have pointed out the possibility of damage to the epidermis if this abrasive cleaning is carried out too vigorously and roughly.

For those who nevertheless decide to use these preparations, this type of cleansing should not be carried out more than once weekly, since the defensive properties of the skin may be affected if the outer layers are removed. Massaging and rubbing these preparations into the skin must be done with the utmost care and gentleness, and in strict accordance with the manufacturer's instructions.

Summary

- Cleansing creams and emulsions offer another means of cleaning the face, but hold no significant advantage over soap and water.
- They should not be used as moisturizers.
- They may be recommended for people removing oily make-up that is water-resistant.
- They may be recommended for people with delicate skin, since the cleansing substances they contain are relatively delicate compared with other types of soaps. However, they must be rinsed off with water, and not just wiped off with a paper tissue or cloth.

7

Facial cleansing masks

Contents   Overview • Functions of a facial mask •   Masks that rinse off and masks
that peel off • 'Absorbent' masks that rinse off • Masks that peel off • 'Exotic' facial
masks • Possible undesirable effects from facial cleansing masks

Overview

The use of facial masks represents a unique approach to cleaning the face and
skin care: the preparation is applied to the skin as a relatively thick layer, and
then removed some time later, usually 15–30 minutes. Note that the facial
mask does not represent an essential technique of skin care. The effects
achieved by facial masks can all be achieved by simpler means, such as washing the face with soap and water, applying moisturizing creams or using
astringent preparations. Nevertheless, facial masks do have certain advantages, which are discussed in this chapter.

Functions of a facial mask

- **Effective cleansing of the skin**, while removing the outer parts of the
  keratinous layer. This type of thorough cleansing, in fact, has a certain
  'peeling' effect, but it is extremely superficial and the degree of peeling is
  negligible compared with the medical procedure of skin peeling as carried
  out by an experienced physician (see Chapter 22 on chemical peeling).
- **Moisturizing the skin**, thereby giving it a smooth, moist appearance –
  provided that the mask contains moisturizers. After using a facial mask,
  the skin becomes slightly swollen, which has the effect of temporarily
  smoothing out fine wrinkles. This effect of skin moisturization is achieved
  by virtue of the occlusive effect of the facial mask, which becomes more
  effective the more moisturizing substances the mask contains.
- **Treatment of acne** – provided the mask is designed for that purpose, and
  contains the appropriate ingredients.
- **Improvement of the overall feeling of well-being**: through the perception
  that the facial skin is being 'coddled' and the feeling of calmness and
  tranquillity while the mask is on the face. In addition, removal of the mask
  is followed by a pleasant, fresh and clean feeling; and usually there is a

sensory effect of 'tautness', resulting from the drying out of the mask on the face, which is even more pronounced if the mask contains astringents.

Note: A facial mask does not 'nourish' the skin. It cannot 'smooth out' wrinkles (other than the temporary 'smoothing' due to skin moisturization). As part of the vigorous marketing and advertising of these products, claims are made to the effect that a facial mask can, for example 'stimulate the blood flow to the skin'. In fact, simple physical or sporting activities will stimulate blood flow in the body and skin much more effectively than will a facial mask – not to mention all the other advantages of physical exercise.

Masks that rinse off and masks that peel off

Masks that rinse off are removed from the skin by rinsing with lukewarm or warm water:

- **absorbent masks** are based on insoluble powders, or natural clay and mud (see below);
- 'gel masks' contain ingredients such as tragacanth;
- some of the masks that are rinsed off are not actually masks, but rather a mixture of moisturizing agents or cleansing agents (or a combination of both) that are marketed, for commercial reasons, as 'facial masks'.

Masks that are peeled off are made of rubbery substances, such as:

- vinyl-based substances (such as polyvinyl alcohol)
- rubber-based substances: latex or other natural rubber compounds

As these masks dry on the skin, they harden and form a thin, flexible, usually transparent sheet on the skin. In this case, the mask is not removed by rinsing with water, but is peeled off the face.

With both masks that are rinsed off and those that are peeled off, it is important that the time for which they remain on the face is in accordance with the manufacturer's instructions. The mask is usually removed 15–30 minutes after application.

In spite of the schematic division into masks that are rinsed off and those that are peeled off, this distinction is not clear-cut. Masks can be made that contain a mixture of ingredients, such as clay (used in masks that are rinsed off) with rubber components (used in masks that are peeled off). Hydrocolloid substances (such as carboxymethyl cellulose) may be added to any type of mask. The final composition of the mask determines whether it can be rinsed off or peeled off.

'Absorbent' masks that rinse off

The basic ingredient of these masks is powder, which is made up of inorganic substances such as zinc oxide, titanium dioxide, kaolin, calamine, and others.

Other masks in this group are based on processed clay and natural mud. Before the mask is applied to the face, the powder is mixed in accordance with the manufacturer's instructions, with water, milk, various fruit or vegetable juices, other extracts, or any liquid specified in the instructions. These masks are also available in the form of a 'paste', in which the powder has already been mixed by the manufacturer. Usually some liquid such as propylene glycol, with a small amount of soap, has to be added, to make it easier to remove the mask from the face.

These masks usually absorb fats from the skin, and are recommended for people with oily skin.

The material is gently applied to the face, and left in place in accordance with the manufacturer's instructions, for some 15–30 minutes. It is then rinsed off with soap and water.

Masks that peel off

These masks do not absorb fats from the skin, as do powder- or clay-based masks. The major effect of these masks is to prevent the evaporation of water from the skin's surface. As a result, the amount of moisture in the skin increases, as long as the mask is on the face.

These masks are recommended for women with relatively dry facial skin.

When these masks are used in a cosmetics salon, a thin layer of gauze can be placed under the mask. This allows the ingredients of the mask to coat the client's skin (since they pass through the gaps in the gauze material), while at the same time allowing the mask to be removed quickly and efficiently in one piece.

The steps in this treatment are shown in the illustrations.

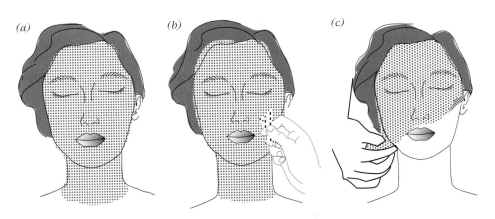

(a) A piece of gauze soaked in water is placed over the face. (b) The mask is applied to the face on top of the gauze. (c) After the required treatment time, the gauze is lifted and rolled up off the face, taking the mask with it.

'Exotic' facial masks

In addition to the types of masks discussed above, other sorts of masks are used in various health resorts and cosmetic clinics, each place having its own 'speciality'. The masks used are, for example, various mud masks (depending on the soil composition of the region), and masks containing beeswax, seaweed extracts or extracts of a wide variety of plants. In general, a wide range of cosmetic ingredients can be added to any type of mask. There is no scientific proof that any of the components of these 'exotic' masks have any advantage in terms of skin care. Furthermore, facial masks may not be very useful in helping cosmetic or other ingredients penetrate into the skin, since they are only on the skin for a relatively short time.

Facial masks for acne

Another type of facial mask is that used in the treatment of acne. These masks are based on:

- substances that absorb oil from the skin
- the incorporation of active ingredients that are used for treating acne, such as sulfur or benzoyl peroxide

These masks may well be an effective adjunct, supplementing other acne treatments.

Possible undesirable effects from facial cleansing masks

Facial cleansing masks may cause:

- skin irritation, which is usually due to an allergic reaction to one or more components of the mask;
- skin infection.

These complications are more likely to occur from the use of masks of dubious origin. The risks of such problems are much less when using masks from a reputable cosmetics manufacturer. In general, before using any mask, one should establish that the client is not allergic to any of its ingredients.

Note: Following the use of a mask, and after it has been rinsed off, moisturizing cream should be applied to the face. This is because a facial mask tends to cause slight superficial 'peeling' of the outermost layers of the skin. Hence it is important to avoid exposure to wind, sun or polluted air after removing a facial cleansing mask. It seems absurd for someone who has just undergone thorough cleansing of her facial skin to go out into a polluted street, full of exhaust fumes. It is wise to wait a reasonable time, until the skin has had a chance to rebuild a protective oily layer.

8

Skin ageing and its modulation

Contents Overview • Skin and age: chronological ageing • Photoageing: ageing of the skin due to sun exposure • Major characteristics of skin ageing • Modulation of skin ageing

Overview

Unfortunately, we are too familiar with the ageing process of the skin. Young individuals with soft, smooth and supple skin become aware, with the passage of time, of signs of ageing: the development and deepening of wrinkles, appearance of age spots and loosening of the skin. These changes occur in all layers of the skin. They can be classified as follows:

1 Changes due to the natural ageing process: **chronological ageing**. Skin ageing is the natural expression of an individual's age. Yet, people of identical chronological age may appear to have younger- or older-looking skin. Genetic factors have a great impact on determining skin quality over time. There is a combination of genetic factors – for example:

   • better innate durability
   • hormonal mechanisms
   • the fact that thicker skin tends to wrinkle less

2 Changes due to **environmental factors**; the leading factor here is **solar radiation**. These changes appear, of course, in areas of the body exposed to the sun. Prolonged exposure to cold, wind and environmental pollutants such as smog may also cause cumulative damage to skin.

   The desire to preserve a youthful appearance has led to the development of a myriad of cosmetic products, marketed with labels such as 'prevents skin ageing' and 'removes wrinkles'. Not all of these products are based on biological reasoning that supports the advertising claims. Most 'before and after' photographs reflect the photographer's technical skill rather than the product's effectiveness.
   This chapter reviews the skin ageing process, possible preventive measures, and corrective methods that have proven to be effective.

Skin and age: chronological ageing

The following changes occur with the natural passage of time. They appear in all areas of the body, regardless of exposure to the sun. They include:

- degeneration of elastin fibres
- degeneration of collagen fibres
- thinning of the skin

Elastin fibres
Thin, functioning elastin fibres of the skin undergo a degenerative process, gradually becoming lumps of fibres of poor quality. The changes in the elastin fibres are the major cause of the development of wrinkles and the loss of skin elasticity.

Collagen fibres
In addition to the degeneration of elastin fibres, there is a gradual degeneration and reduction in the amount of collagen fibres. This causes a decline in skin strength, with subsequent loosening of skin.

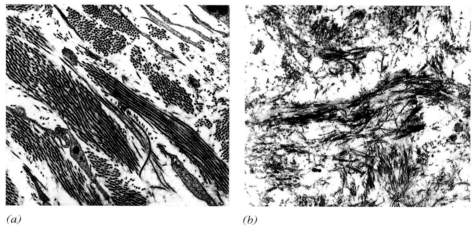

(a)   *(b)*

(a) Collagen fibres in the dermis of 'young skin'. (b) Collagen fibres in the dermis of 'old skin'.

Thinning of the skin
In general, starting at approximately 45 years of age, there is a gradual thinning of all skin layers, including the epidermis, dermis and subcutaneous layers. This process is more pronounced in a woman's than in a man's skin. There is also a gradual flattening of the wavy attachment between the epidermis and dermis.

The subcutaneous fatty layer becomes thinner. Loss of the fatty layer is more prominent in certain areas: face, hands and calves. This process of degeneration and waning of tissue is called **atrophy**.

(a) 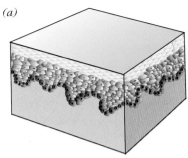 *(b)*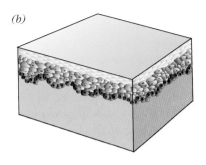

Flattening of the attachment between epidermis and dermis in older skin (b), compared with the wavy attachment in younger skin (a).

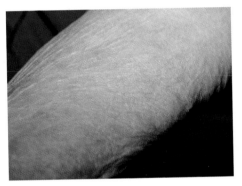

Extremely thin atrophic skin.

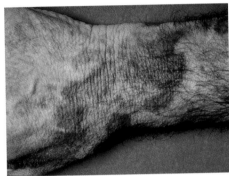

Bruise (local haemorrhage) in an older man's forearm.

All of the above changes cause the appearance of wrinkles and loss of skin elasticity. The loss of the skin's strength and thickness causes the skin, and the layers beneath it, to become more vulnerable. With advancing age, there is a tendency to develop local haemorrhages as a result of minimal trauma: this is termed 'easy bruisability'. It occurs as a result of the poor quality of the skin, as well as the increased fragility of the blood vessels.

Additional changes that appear in the skin with age
With increasing age:

- the skin becomes drier;
- there are changes in hair growth;
- there are changes in pigmentation;
- the sebaceous glands become enlarged.

Dry skin
This results from a gradual decline in the activity of the sebaceous glands. This decline is apparent after menopause in women, and at a later age in men. The sebum produced by sebaceous glands forms a fine lipid layer over the skin surface. This lipid layer serves as a barrier preventing evaporation of water

from the skin. A decrease in the production of sebum will therefore cause the skin to become drier.

There is also a decrease in the ability of skin to retain its water content.

Extremely dry skin in older individuals may become a nuisance and may cause severe itching. The medical term for extreme dryness is **xerosis**.

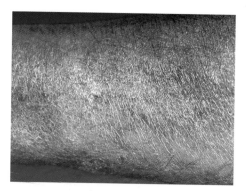

Dry, cracked, xerotic skin.

Changes in hair growth
Thinning of hair appears in most areas of the body. As an individual ages, the quantity of hair decreases, as well as its thickness. However, the reverse process occurs in certain areas, such as the ears and eyebrows in men: hair that was previously unnoticeable in these areas becomes thicker and darker, posing a significant aesthetic problem.

Loss of melanocytes (melanin-producing cells)
With increasing age, there is a decline in the number of melanocytes in the skin, which results in a decrease in the production of melanin. The skin tone, in general, becomes lighter. The decrease in melanin means that the skin's function as a barrier against the sun's radiation is less effective.

On the other hand, in areas of the skin that are exposed to the sun, there may be a proliferation of melanocytes. This will be manifested by the appearance of darker spots on the skin.

Enlargement of sebaceous glands
In certain areas, despite a decrease in the amount of sebum produced by the skin, the sebaceous glands increase in size. As a result, the skin's pores may widen. The glands enlarge and may appear to the naked eye as flat yellowish blemishes, up to 3 mm wide, upon the skin's surface.

Because of the high density of sebaceous glands on the nose, this process causes gradual thickening, enlargement and a general change in appearance of the nose.

Photoageing: ageing of the skin due to sun exposure

Exposure to the sun is the primary environmental cause of skin damage, along with other external factors such as prolonged exposure to cold and wind. As previously stated, the major factor in the formation of wrinkles and loss of skin firmness is the destruction of elastin fibres. Degeneration of these fibres, which occurs naturally in gradually ageing skin, is intensified by prolonged exposure to the sun. The elastin degenerates as exposure to the sun continues.

Chronological ageing, which occurs naturally with the passage of time, differs in its presentation compared with photoageing. For example, in photoageing, more cells are formed in the epidermis, which thickens in an irregular pattern. This is in stark contrast to the thinning of the epidermis, which occurs during normal ageing, in skin not exposed to the sun.

Additional characteristics of photoageing are:

- uneven pigmentation;
- the appearance of 'age spots', the medical term for which is **solar lentigines**;
- the possible development of skin tumours, typical of photoageing;
- the appearance of dilated blood vessels in the skin – these are called **telangiectases**.

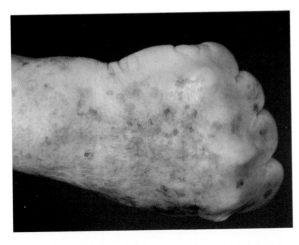

Solar lentigines ('age spots').

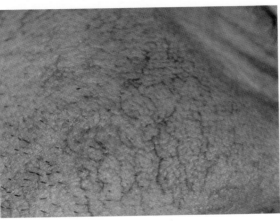

Telangiectases in facial skin.

Chronological ageing	Photoageing
Thin, atrophic skin	An irregular pattern of thicker skin; an increase in the number of epidermal cells
Degeneration of collagen and elastin fibres	Accelerated degeneration of collagen and elastin fibres
Possible development of skin tumours	Possible development of skin tumours, which are typical of photoageing
Lighter skin due to decline in melanin production	Uneven pigmentation: appearance of 'age spots' (solar lentigines)
Additional features: • drier skin • changes in hair growth • enlargement of sebaceous glands	Additional features: • telangiectases (dilated blood vessels in the skin)

How can one demonstrate the differences between chronological changes in the skin and those caused by sun exposure?

Compare, in a middle-aged individual, the skin on the inner part of the upper arm – skin that is not exposed to the sun – with that on the back of the hand – which is constantly exposed:

- The skin on the inner arm is smooth and looks younger.
- The elasticity of the skin on the outer hand is significantly reduced. The skin is wrinkled and characterized by irregular pigmentation.

Older people may show the first signs of skin lesions and tumours, depending on their personal history of sun exposure.

Major characteristics of skin ageing

Degeneration of elastin and collagen fibres occurs, as previously discussed, both in chronological skin ageing and in photoageing. These changes lead to the appearance of:

- fine wrinkles
- pronounced and deepened lines of expression
- skin sagging

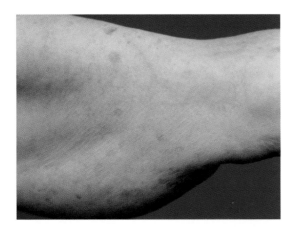

Inner arm.

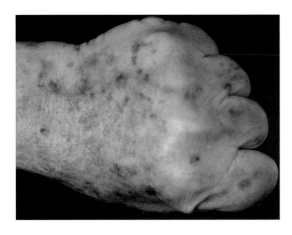

Outer hand of the same person after prolonged exposure to the sun.

Fine wrinkles

With the decline in quantity and quality of the elastin fibres, the skin loosens. It loses its elasticity and its ability to return to its original state after stretching. When the elastin fibres degenerate, the skin gradually acquires a large number of fine wrinkles – everyone over the age of 75 years has wrinkling over their skin's surface.

Deepening of expressive lines

The facial muscles are attached directly to the skin. The facial region is relatively poor in its subcutaneous fat content. Thus every facial expression causes folding of the skin, because muscles can contract, but skin cannot.

In the young, facial expressions disappear when the muscles are relaxed, because elastin fibres function properly in the skin. But when the muscles contract beneath degenerated elastic tissue, fine wrinkles appear. They remain even when the face is passive and devoid of all expression.

These wrinkles are formed uniquely in each person. Expressive habits are formed late in childhood, and remain subconsciously throughout life. Eventually they form an individual pattern of facial expressions. With time, these facial lines become permanent, and may lead to a misinterpretation of moods or feelings. These lines may impart an expression of fatigue, anger or depression that in itself does not necessarily represent the individual's actual mood.

In observing people's expressions, it is easy to understand the formation of wrinkles. For example, when the eyebrows are raised, horizontal expression lines are formed on the forehead.

It should be noted that expressions also affect the formation of fine wrinkles. One can observe the wrinkling of the fine skin of the eyelids when squinting or raising the eyebrows.

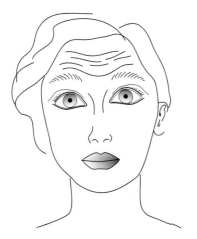 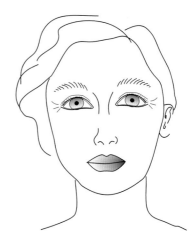

Raising eyebrows forms horizontal expression lines on the forehead.   *Squinting causes lines, termed 'crow's feet', at the outer edges of the eyes.*

Loosening and sagging of the skin
A combination of decreased skin thickness and strength, as well as a decrease in the thickness of the subcutaneous fatty layer, causes loosening and sagging of the skin. Gravity pulls the slack skin even further. In addition, bone loss begins at an age of approximately 60 years. Resorption of the lower jaw bone and cheekbones may further contribute to the appearance of loose facial skin.

Muscle hypotonia
Loss of muscle tension imparts a loose appearance to the facial skin.

Modulation of skin ageing

The process of skin ageing is not fully understood. Currently, there is no definitive way to prevent this process. However, there are practical measures that can be taken to minimize the effects:

• minimize sun exposure

- avoid smoking
- prevent unnecessary stretching of the skin
- change personal expressive habits, if necessary
- use hormone replacement therapy for post-menopausal women
- use certain topical products
- lead a healthier emotional and physical lifestyle

Avoiding sun exposure

Exposure to the sun causes:

- destructive damage to the elastin fibres in the skin
- induction of tumours, both benign and malignant
- changes in skin pigmentation

Excessive exposure to solar radiation must be avoided. Moderate limitations of time spent outdoors and the use of hats and sunscreens are recommended.

Note: Sunglasses prevent damage caused by the penetration of ultraviolet rays to the eyes. In addition, they prevent the inevitable response of squinting that occurs in sunlight. Such prolonged, repeated squinting may accelerate the appearance of 'crow's feet'-type wrinkles, so the use of sunglasses is highly recommended.

Photoageing is discussed in detail in Chapter 10 on sun and the skin.

Smoking

Smoking has health as well as aesthetic effects on the skin. We shall not elaborate on other major health hazards caused by smoking, such as vascular, lung, heart, brain and other diseases.

The characteristics of a smoker's face are well recognized. Chronic smokers have pale, yellowish-grey skin. Deep lines typically appear radially from the upper and lower lips, and laterally from the eyes. There is relative skin thickening between these wrinkles.

Causes of skin damage due to smoking

- Nicotine causes vascular constriction that decreases the normal nourishment of the skin by the blood.
- Additional toxic products in the smoke may cause damage to external layers of the skin (through direct contact).
- Absorption of these toxic products and their introduction to the skin through the circulation may damage the collagen and elastic fibres.
- Smoke may also cause dryness and irritation. If prolonged, this may damage the skin.
- Exposure to smoke is irritating to the eyes. This causes repeated squinting, which results in the appearance of 'crow's feet'-type wrinkles.

Additional aesthetic deterrents of smoking

- Staining of fingers and teeth.
- After plastic surgery (such as a face lift or peeling procedures), the healing is delayed, and is not as effective as it is for non-smokers. This is probably due to damage to blood vessels.

In 1992, the *American Journal of Epidemiology* published an article entitled: 'Does cigarette smoking make you ugly and old?' The answer, in short, is yes!

Preventing unnecessary stretching of the skin

Pregnancy can serve as an example of this issue: gradual stretching of the abdominal skin during pregnancy results in an increase in surface area. Excess skin is formed by its gradual expansion. After delivery, the skin may appear more slack and loose. In younger women, the skin is more supple; therefore the actual effect of pregnancy on the skin is minimal.

Tissue expanders – What does stretching of the skin result in?

The use of tissue expanders in plastic surgery also illustrates this concept. A tissue expander is a bag or balloon made of inert materials, and filled with water.

This procedure is utilized in regions where there is an absence of skin. It is performed in various medical conditions, including traumatic injury, burns and certain diseases. The surgeon requires supplementary skin to cover areas devoid of skin. In order to obtain additional skin, the expander is transplanted below the patient's skin, adjacent to the deficient area. This results in expansion of the healthy skin, which is later used to cover skinless areas.

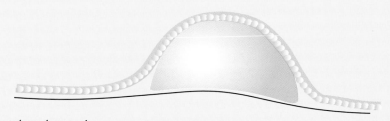

A transplanted expander.

Over a period of several weeks, additional water is injected into the transplanted expander, increasing its volume. As a result, the overlying skin is stretched, and its surface gradually expands.

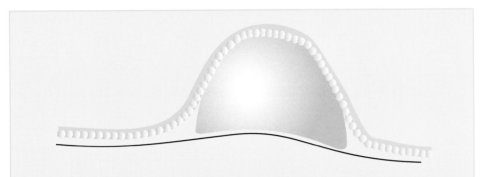

Volume increase of the expander, with subsequent expansion of the skin surface above.

Next the expander is removed from the patient's body. After removal, the excess skin remains loose, and can be stretched to cover adjacent areas, as necessary.

This is the main idea in using tissue expanders: a gradual stretching of the skin causes an increase in the skin's surface area, with the production of excess skin.

The cosmetic significance is that any stretching of the skin, whether gradual or repeated, causes the skin surface to expand. When this process is not intended for medical purposes, the skin is not utilized for covering adjacent surfaces. This skin remains loose, slack and wrinkled. The cosmetic implications are clear: **unnecessary stretching of the skin should be avoided**.

Unnecessary facial expressions, as detailed later in the text, cause repeated stretching of the skin, and should be avoided. Training and exercising of the facial muscles can cause unnecessary stretching of the skin. It is a myth that these exercises are beneficial to facial skin. As previously explained, such exercises may actually accelerate the process of wrinkling. Even when one is applying facial cosmetic products, this must be done gently to avoid stretching of the skin.

The same principle holds for **abrupt changes in weight**. Extreme weight gain accompanied by an increase in the amount of subcutaneous fat causes stretching of the skin above the thickened fatty layer. With weight loss, skin that was previously stretched becomes slack, and the excess skin becomes wrinkled and loose. So a balanced diet should be followed, in order to avoid repeated weight gain and loss.

And one more comment...

It has been suggested that sleeping on one side causes stretching of the face in certain directions due to gravity, so diagonal wrinkles are formed on the cheeks and forehead. Therefore sleeping in a supine position may be recommended. There is some degree of biological logic in this argument, but it is difficult to substantiate. No medical studies on this issue have been conducted. Because of the complexities involved, and the long periods of follow-up required, it is unlikely that such studies will take place.

Changes in personal habits

As previously described, when observing people during animated conversation, it is easy to see why expressive lines are formed.

Facial expressions and wrinkles: unilateral paralysis

There is additional proof that facial expressions can cause wrinkles. In people with unilateral paralysis, after a number of years, the paralysed side fo the face appears 'younger'. In contrast, the side of the face with normal movement and expression gains lines with time.

What can be done?

Certainly, the object is not to develop a 'poker face', nor is the intent to achieve total lack of facial movement. Normal expressions and expressive lines impart unique facial characteristics. One's personality, characteristics and history are defined in the expressions and lines of one's face.

Some suggest that excessively exaggerated facial expressions be avoided during normal conversation in order to prevent the formation of unnecessary expressive lines over time.

Hormone replacement therapy (HRT)

During the reproductive years in women, **oestrogen** is released from the ovaries. This hormone significantly contributes to the 'young', fresh, soft appearance of the skin. With the approach of the menopause, there is a decrease in the level of oestrogen released from the ovaries. Therefore, as well as the general effects of the menopause, there is also a progressive damage to the appearance of the skin and its function.

Hormone replacement therapy (**HRT**) is today commonly prescribed by gynaecologists. The replacement therapy can be taken orally, as tablets, or as hormone-containing patches that adhere to the skin. The advantages of this therapy include prevention of hot flushes, prevention of dryness of the vagina, and a decrease in symptoms of depression and fatigue, as well as decreases in cardiovascular disease and osteoporosis.

Several studies have documented the effects on the skin of HRT with oestrogen. This treatment has been reported to prevent, to a certain extent, the decrease of collagen content in the skin that appears after menopause. In addition, HRT may delay the undesirable accumulation of subcutaneous fat in various areas of the body that accompanies the ageing process.

The use of hormone preparations must be adjusted for each woman according to her specific medical profile, and a physician should be consulted in all cases.

Note that several topical cosmetic products contain hormones, and therefore are advertised as having 'anti-ageing' qualities. These products contain oestrogens in very low concentrations. Because of the minimal amount of hormones they contain, these products remain categorized as cosmetics, and are not labelled as drugs. It has not been confirmed scientifically that these hormone-containing products have any beneficial effect on the skin. Most dermatologists do not recommend them. This is in stark contrast to HRT (where the hormone is in higher concentrations, and is absorbed into the blood, being taken either as a tablet or as a hormone-containing patch), which is generally accepted as benefiting post-menopausal women. HRT is also recommended for most post-menopausal women from an aesthetic point of view.

Use of certain topical products
Skin ageing, whether chronological or sun-induced, was previously considered to be irreversible. In the past few years, a number of new products that can affect the ageing process have been developed, revolutionizing cosmetic dermatology. These include:

- retinoic acid
- alpha-hydroxy acids

These products are discussed in detail in Chapters 16 and 17 respectively. Other products (including preparations containing topical vitamins) are detailed in Chapter 15 on active ingredients in cosmetic preparations.

Until recently, products advertised as effective against wrinkles were simply based on increasing skin moisture. Moisturizers increase the water content of the skin. They give the skin a healthier, swollen appearance, blurring and diminishing the appearance of fine wrinkles – although only temporarily.

Moisturizers – Do they prevent skin ageing?
Certain moisturizing products are marketed as having 'age-reversing' and 'anti-ageing' qualities. However, moisturizers have never been established in the prevention of the skin ageing process – whether caused by advanced age or by sun exposure. Nevertheless, the use of moisturizing products does have benefits.

- It can prevent skin damage caused by excessive dryness.
- An oily layer on the skin surface can protect it from exposure to various environmental factors such as soot particles, dirt and dust.
- As previously stated, when skin is well moisturized, it appears temporarily smoother and more refreshed. Since it is slightly swollen, there is flattening and virtual fading of fine wrinkles. The pores appear somewhat smaller, because the skin surrounding them is distended. This temporary improvement is exploited by advertisers, who claim that various moisturizing products have 'anti-ageing' qualities.

Protecting the skin from environmental factors and preventing damage caused by dryness are highly significant, and without a doubt minimize deterioration in the appearance and quality of facial skin.

Moisturizers are recommended for dry and normal skin, but not for oily skin. Details are given in Chapter 4.

Leading a physically and emotionally healthy lifestyle
A healthy lifestyle will significantly improve one's general health. This includes the skin, a unique organ of the human body. The term 'healthy lifestyle' includes:

- physical activity
- regular sleeping hours
- a healthy, balanced diet
- a healthy mental and emotional state

These will affect the body as a whole, and the skin specifically.

Physical activity

As a rule, physical activity bestows well-being. During physical activity, there is an increase of blood flow to the skin, creating a rosy/red colour. In the long run, this may also improve the skin's texture.

Sleep

After a sleepless night, red eyes and dark shadows around them are a familiar sight – this should be avoided. It is reasonable to assume that, in the long run, sleeplessness may cause cumulative damage to the skin texture.

A healthy, balanced diet

The significance of remaining at a steady weight was stated previously. One should avoid fluctuations in weight. In addition, various nutritional deficiencies are closely linked to dermatological diseases.

For example, severe vitamin C deficiency causes **scurvy**. This disease is manifested by the appearance of haemorrhages in the skin; the gums swell and bleed, with eventual loss of teeth; the body's ability to heal wounds is also adversely affected. Another example is **pellagra**, a disease caused by vitamin B3 deficiency. The appearance of inflamed rashes in areas exposed to the sun is typical of this disease.

Other nutritional deficiencies may manifest themselves by various skin lesions. These include lack of other vitamins, proteins, fatty acids, and trace elements such as iron or zinc. Although these diseases will only manifest themselves with extreme deficiencies, it is reasonable to assume that persistent minimal deficiencies may result in accumulative damage, and should be avoided. So a balanced diet, composed of all the food groups and vitamin requirements, is highly recommended.

In the last decade, much attention has been devoted to vitamins functioning as **anti-oxidants**. These include:

- vitamin C
- beta-carotene
- vitamin E (alpha-tocopherol)

The assumption is that these products entrap the **oxygen free radicals** that cause damage to the body tissues.

What are oxygen free radicals?

Oxygen free radicals are by-products formed by the chemical changes that the oxygen molecule undergoes. They are produced naturally and regularly in the body's tissues. The production of these free radicals in the body is much higher in response to several situations, for example exposure to sunlight, X-rays, smoking and environmental pollutants.

Free radicals damage cell membranes and DNA, and alter various biochemical compounds within the cells. It seems that they play a significant role in the development of heart and blood vessel diseases and the induction of malignancies.

Scientists believe that oxygen free radicals enhance the process of ageing in various body systems, by their gradual and cumulative effect.

Vitamin E, vitamin C and beta-carotene are able to entrap oxygen free radicals. Studies have been conducted in order to establish whether dietary supplements of these vitamins can decrease the incidence of malignancies and cardiovascular disease. Despite publications defending this statement, it is still a controversial issue. Whether or not supplementary vitamins improve the skin's quality and delay the ageing process has not been established, either.

A healthy mental and emotional state

The relationship between mental health and skin health has been well documented for thousands of years. A person's mental and emotional state may be externalized, expressed on the skin – going pale or blushing for example. Emotions, such as rage, anxiety or fear, cause a drop in the temperature of the fingertips. A prolonged state of anxiety may therefore cause damage to the skin texture and its health.

Many diseases, including various skin diseases, are linked to mental stress, and may be exacerbated following a deterioration in the patient's mental health – for example acne, atopic dermatitis, psoriasis and other diseases. Expressive worry lines and depressed facial expressions are established and etched gradually, over years, on the face.

We shall not elaborate on this subject; ample literature has been published regarding this issue. In brief, it may be helpful to lead a happy lifestyle – it certainly cannot hurt.

9

Acne

Overview

Acne is an inflammatory disease of the hair follicles and their associated sebaceous glands. It is related primarily to hormonal changes that occur during adolescence. In most cases, acne appears at 12–14 years of age. Since sexual development begins earlier in girls than in boys, acne appears earlier in girls. Acne may become quite severe after a number of years: between the ages of 15–19, following which there is a gradual improvement and disappearance of the lesions, usually in the mid-20s. Acne can persist, in a minority of patients, into the 40s. The afflicted person should be aware of the fact that the problem may last more than 10 years, and treatment may be necessary from time to time during this period.

Lesions in acne

Acne is characterized by the appearance of:

- **open comedones (blackheads)**
- **closed comedones (whiteheads)**

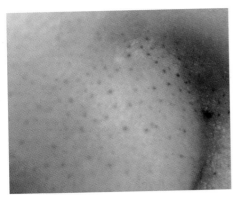

Open comedones (blackheads).

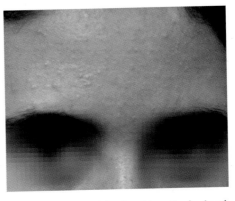

Closed comedones (whiteheads) on the forehead.

Note that the correct medical term is 'comedo' (plural 'comedones'). However, the term 'comedone' is commonly used as well – and we shall do so here.

The comedone is the basic, primary lesion of acne. Other lesions that appear in acne represent various degrees of inflammation, and include the following:

- **Papules** are small, raised lesions, up to 0.5 cm in diameter, usually pink/red in colour.
- **Pustules** are lesions containing pus.

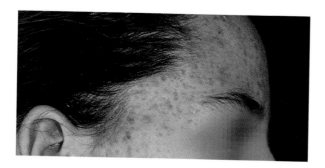

Papules.

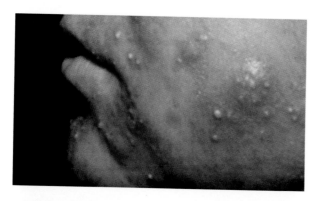

Pustules.

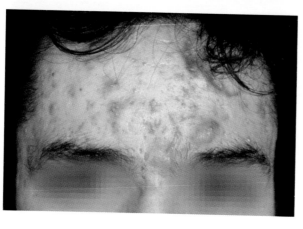

Nodules.

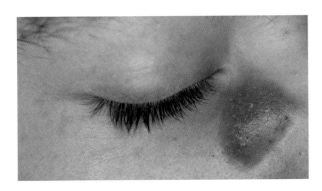

Cyst.

- **Nodules** are inflammatory swellings that, in comparison to papules, are located deeper under the skin. When large, a nodule may change the contour of the skin, thus creating a bulge.
- **Cysts** are closed spaces under the skin's surface, containing liquid or semi-solid material.

The basis for the appearance of acne lesions

Structure of the hair follicle and the sebaceous gland
In order to understand why acne lesions appear and the reason for their development, one should be familiar with the microscopic structure of the skin, the hair follicle and the sebaceous gland.

A **hair follicle** is an elongated tube-like structure, out of which the hair grows – as shown in the diagram. Each hair follicle has one or more **sebaceous**

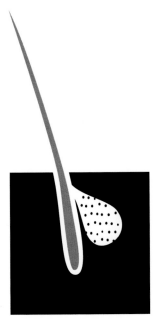

Hair follicle with a hair growing out of it, and the sebaceous gland attached to it.

glands attached to it. The sebaceous gland secretes **sebum**, which is an oily substance that coats the skin and hair. Sebum is not secreted directly onto the surface of the skin, but into the hair follicle, from where it reaches the skin surface. The length and width of each hair are not necessarily correlated with the size of the sebaceous gland whose contents drain to the same hair follicle. For example, on the skin of a woman's face, or on the nose, sebaceous glands are relatively very large, while hairs in this area are barely discernible. When the hair is small, and the opening of the hair follicle is wide and gaping, it looks as though there is a tiny pore on the skin's surface.

Sebaceous glands are distributed throughout the skin of the whole body, except for the palms and soles. They are deeper and more numerous on the face, upper chest and upper back. These areas are indeed more prone to acne.

Primary lesions in acne: closed comedones and open comedones

There are two main reasons for the appearance of the primary acne lesions (the closed comedone and the open comedone).

- an increase in the number of cells in the hair follicle, which results in an increase of the horny substance (keratin) found in the hair follicle;
- an increase in sebum production by the sebaceous glands.

Normally, cells in the hair follicle replicate steadily and continuously, as do other cells on the skin surface. Similarly, there is a constant, steady secretion of sebum by the sebaceous glands. Under normal circumstances, cells that are shed within the follicle are swept out of the follicle onto the surface of the skin, along with the secreted sebum.

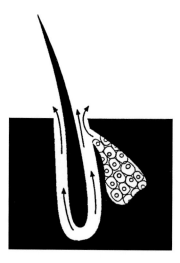

Normally the contents of the skin follicle are swept onto the skin surface.

However, in acne, the replication of cells within the hair follicle is excessive. Within the follicle, there are increasing amounts of oily substances and keratinous (horny) material (originating from the secreted sebum and the accumulation of dead cells), with subsequent difficulty in draining these substances from the follicle to the surface of the skin. With time, these keratinous and oily substances block off the tiny ducts through which the sebum drains to the surface of the skin. In the next stage, the draining duct widens and the sebaceous gland grows larger and wider due to the accumulated material. This process is shown in illustrations 1–4.

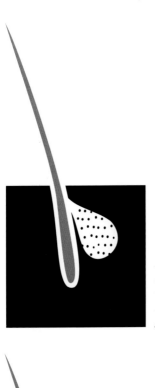

1   Cross-section of a hair follicle: normal sebaceous gland.

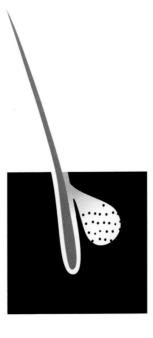

2   The duct leading from the sebaceous gland is blocked by sebum and keratin.

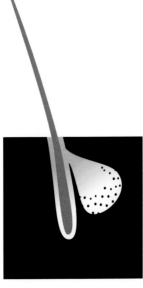

3   The sebum, produced in the sebaceous gland, accumulates behind the area of blockage.

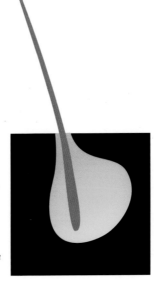

4   The accumulated sebum distends the sebaceous gland and its duct.

As a result of this process, the two basic lesions of acne appear. (Note that at this point these lesions are not yet inflamed.)

Open comedones (blackheads)

These are caused by a widening of the follicle opening owing to the accumulation of dense keratinous material and sebum. The black colour seen in the pore comes from the presence of pigment, which is also found among the substances that plug the opening of the follicle.

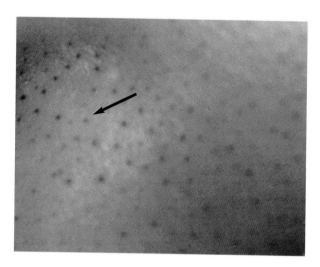

An open comedone (blackhead).

Closed comedones (whiteheads)

These occur when the follicle's opening remains closed. Underneath the opening of the follicle, the dense keratinous material and sebum accumulate. A closed comedone, in itself, is not an inflammatory lesion, but it is the initial lesion from which the various inflammatory lesions in acne may develop.

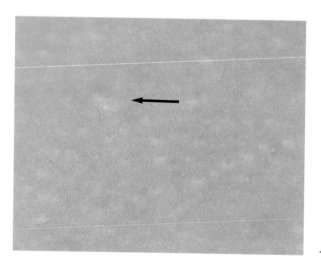

A closed comedone (whitehead).

Inflammatory lesions of acne

As already pointed out, the inflammatory lesions of acne develop from the closed comedone (whitehead), which is a closed space filled with sebum, fatty substances, compressed keratinous material and remnants of dead cells. These conditions permit a proliferation of bacteria naturally found within the hair follicles and on the skin surface. However, within the closed comedone, bacteria in the depths of the follicle enjoy ideal conditions for proliferation: a nutritional environment rich in fats (sebum) and without oxygen, within the enclosed space. The bacteria replicate rapidly and excrete substances that induce an inflammatory reaction. This bacterial action produces the inflammatory lesions in acne. These lesions were listed earlier in the chapter, and we now review them in detail, together with schematic illustrations.

Papules

These are the primary inflammatory lesions. A papule is a lesion that is usually smaller than 0.5 cm in diameter. It is raised above the skin's surface. As a result of the inflammatory process in acne, it acquires a pink to red colour.

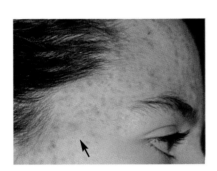

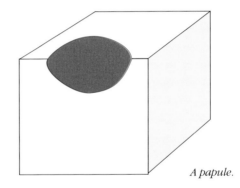

A papule.

Pustules

If the follicle's space becomes filled with pus, the result is a pustule. Pustules are tiny spaces containing pus. Their colour ranges from white/yellow to orange/green. Puncturing a pustule releases its liquid pus content.

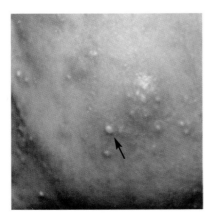

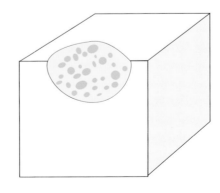

A pustule.

Nodules

When more and more keratinous remnants and sebum accumulate within the follicle, it becomes larger and deeper, resulting in a nodule. A nodule is an inflamed swelling located deeper in the skin compared with a papule. The distinction between a papule and a nodule can be made by feeling the lesion with the fingers.

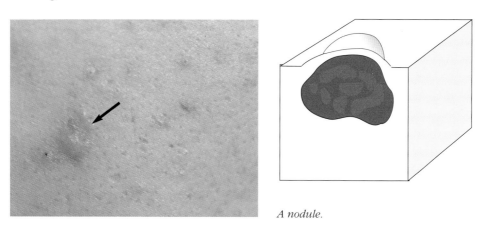

A nodule.

Cysts

When the hair follicle becomes filled with a liquid substance, the result is a cyst. A cyst is a fluid-containing space within the skin. By carefully feeling a cyst, one can feel the presence of the liquid substance contained within it.

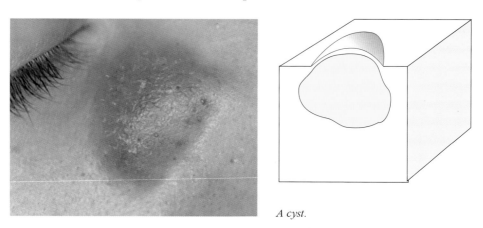

A cyst.

Diet and acne

In most cases, diet has no influence on acne. However, a few dietary recommendations may be given for acne patients.

Sensitivity to particular foods

Although for most patients, there is no association between dietary factors and acne, there are exceptional cases where a certain food does cause acne to appear within days of its ingestion. If there is an obvious correlation between consumption of this food and acne then the patient should avoid that specific food.

Milk products and acne
An acne patient being treated with antibiotics of the tetracycline group should avoid milk products while taking these drugs. After ingestion of milk products, one should wait at least two hours before taking these antibiotics. For acne patients who are not taking tetracyclines, there is no special reason to avoid milk products.

Alternative medical treatments associated with diet
In the standard medical literature, there is no proof that alternative therapies are effective in acne. Nevertheless, these forms of treatment are usually harmless. Therefore, if an acne sufferer is interested in alternative therapies (whether or not they involve dietary changes), they can be tried, provided there is no possibility that they will harm his/her health. In any case, these therapies should be used in conjunction with conventional medical acne treatment. In general, nowadays it is quite rare for acne not to improve with conventional medical treatment, taking into account the wide range of treatments currently available.

Facial cleansing

Acne is a process that does not originate from the skin's surface, but from the deeper layers – inside the follicles and the sebaceous glands. Therefore merely cleaning and washing the face cannot solve the problem, since the cause of acne is primarily hormonal. People with clean skin can most definitely develop acne; just as those whose skin is less clean may escape the disease.

However, cleansing may have some positive effect, by rinsing and removing sebum, sweat, dirt and dead cells from the surface of the skin. Removing the oily layer and dirt from the skin's surface may, to some extent, reduce the 'blockages' in the pores, allowing a more effective drainage of the contents of the hair follicles. (By the same token, the exact opposite process – applying oil to an oily skin that is prone to acne and sealing the pores – may aggravate acne). Furthermore, even though the cleansing process does not reach deep into the follicles and the sebaceous glands, it may possibly remove bacteria found on the skin's surface and prevent them from penetrating into the follicles. Surface cleansing of the skin is not supposed to cure a pre-existing comedone – at the most, it may prevent the infection from spreading and may prevent the development of new lesions. That being the case, acne sufferers are advised to wash the face gently, two or three times a day, in order to remove excess dirt, oily substances, bacteria and dead cells from the skin's surface.

Cleansing should be done gently. Vigorous rubbing and scrubbing has no additional benefits, and indeed may worsen the acne by spreading the inflammation to new areas. A relatively mild soap should be used rather than a drying one, since most of the preparations used in the treatment of acne already contain substances that tend to dry the skin. If the skin becomes red, irritated or scaly while using a certain soap, another, more gentle type should be tried.

Soaps

The soaps recommended for acne patients are relatively mild. They do not tend to cause irritant reactions. Another group of soaps used in acne contain antibacterial compounds, in order to act against bacteria that cause acne. These soaps are detailed in Chapter 5 on skin cleansing.

Benzoyl peroxide in acne soaps
Benzoyl peroxide is a common antibacterial compound used in acne, and is found in acne soaps. This peroxide is an oxidant that acts against the bacteria that cause acne. It is found in many acne preparations for application to the skin, and has been found to be effective in the treatment of acne (see below). However, benzoyl peroxide is less efficacious when it is in a soap or other cleansing preparations that are rinsed off shortly after being applied to the skin than when it is in a preparation that is left on the skin for several hours.

Sun and acne

When acne patients are exposed to the sun, the majority show some improvement. About one-fifth of patients will not respond, and in the minority of patients, there is aggravation of the skin lesions. The improvement is related to a certain anti-inflammatory effect of the ultraviolet rays. In addition, tanning may conceal the acne lesions to some extent. However, exposure to the sun's rays may also cause an excess production of keratin and sebum, both on the skin's surface and in the pores, which may, in turn, cause a relative worsening of the acne. Some dermatologists therefore recommend that the face be gently cleansed after being moderately exposed to the sun.

In summary:
- Exposure to the sun should be gradual and moderate.
- If a patient notices an aggravation of acne after exposure to the sun then he/she should avoid such exposure.
- Gentle cleansing of the skin after exposure to the sun may be recommended.
- A non-oily sunscreen that suits the patient's skin should be used. It should be remembered that the use of some oily moisturizers may aggravate the acne.

Note: The above discussion relates to non-inflammatory lesions of acne. While **active inflammatory lesions** of acne are present, it is best to avoid sun exposure, since these lesions sometimes heal by the formation of scars. In general, sun exposure may darken the final colour of scars, including acne scars, thus making them more apparent.

Cosmetics and make-up

Two types of cosmetics may cause acne:

- **Comedogenic** preparations, i.e. substances that encourage the appearance of comedones: in those cases the acne usually appears after using the cosmetic for several months. Comedones begin to appear – both whiteheads and blackheads.
- **Acnegenic** preparations: in these cases, the acne appears in the form of pustules, within one to two weeks of using the formulation.

Usually make-up preparations that are too oily may cause occlusion of the skin's pores, interfering with the normal drainage of sebum secretion, and therefore they have comedogenic or acnegenic potential. In the cosmetics industry, emphasis has been put on the identification of certain ingredients that may reduce acne. Many cosmetics include a label specifying that they are either non-comedogenic or non-acnegenic. In general, cosmetics for women who suffer from acne are designed for use on oily skin. These preparations, as a rule, contain a relatively larger concentration of water (and less oil), and may even contain oil-absorbing substances.

Similarly, there are creams intended for acne treatment in which the medical preparations are combined with colouring ingredients. These can be used simultaneously as make-up. The user can match the colour of the cream to the skin colour by using the proper amount of the colouring ingredient.

Treatment by a cosmetician

The main functions of a cosmetician in treating acne are:

- cleansing of the face
- expressing the contents of the comedones
- instructing patients how to clean and treat the skin

Obviously, this treatment should be carried out together with medical treatment given by a physician.

Note: The part of the cosmetician's treatment described below, namely opening and draining comedones, has no effect on the duration and the general course of the disease. The treatment is aimed at preventing comedones from becoming inflamed or infected, but new comedones will continue to appear. However, appropriate treatment by a cosmetician does produce an immediate cosmetic improvement, with all its psychological benefits.

The stages in treating comedones are:

1 softening the comedones
2 cleaning and sterilizing the skin
3 expressing the contents of the comedones
4 further cleansing of the affected area

Softening the comedones

It is preferable that the patient be given treatment to soften the comedones before draining them. Ideally, this is achieved by the use of creams containing retinoic acid. The cream should be applied to the affected area, daily, for one month, before the cosmetician commences treatment. This preliminary treatment can only be prescribed by a dermatologist.

Alternative methods for softening and loosening the comedones are:

- by steaming;
- applying hot, moist compresses 15 minutes before treatment;
- application of preparations with salicylic acid or sulfur salicylic acid before treatment is given.

Cleaning and sterilizing the skin

This can be achieved using alcohol (70% solution) or any other antiseptic solution.

Expressing the contents of the comedones

There are two ways to achieve this:

- squeezing with the fingertips
- using a **comedone extractor**

Both methods are acceptable, and each has its advocates.

What are the arguments in favour of using a comedone extractor?

Squeezing the comedones with the fingertips, if not done correctly, may result in the contents of the comedone bursting into the surrounding tissue. This may cause inflammation in the area and result in scarring.

These days, with the emergence of HIV and an increase in the incidence of hepatitis B infection, any contact with the blood or secretions of a patient requires the use of gloves. A cosmetician who squeezes comedones with the fingertips must also wear gloves, since the treatment may cause some localized bleeding. However, by wearing gloves, the cosmetician may lose the delicate feeling in the fingertips needed for the treatment, and the whole process becomes awkward and much less efficient.

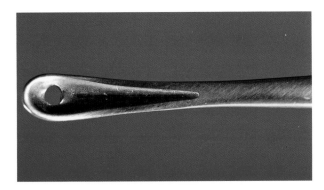

Comedone extractor.

On the other hand, many cosmeticians prefer the old method of squeezing the comedones with the fingertips. They maintain that in fact, the firm vertical pressure that the comedone extractor exerts on the follicle (downwards, towards the deeper layers of the skin), may actually cause the follicle to burst – which, they believe, does not happen when an experienced cosmetician uses the fingertips. Some proponents of this method recommend covering the fingers with a thin layer of cotton-wool soaked in a weak alcohol solution.

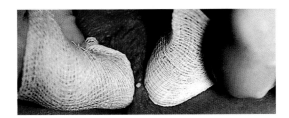

Expressing the contents of a comedone by squeezing with the fingertips.

Note: All the treatments described here must be performed under optimal conditions, with a bright light and a magnifying glass.

How is it done?

- **Open comedone (blackhead)**: This is expressed by applying vertical pressure – gentle, yet steady – pressing downwards around the sides of the lesion. The pressure applied to a comedone ought to push the contents up and out, onto the surface of the skin. If nothing comes out, the fingers should be moved a little bit to a different location around the lesion and the procedure repeated. If fatty material starts to ooze out of the comedone, one should press gently in a few places (using two opposing fingers) until all the contents have come out, or a little bleeding occurs. The extruded material should be wiped from the skin with cotton-wool (not gauze or tissue, which have a rougher consistency than cotton-wool), and the area then wiped again with antiseptic.

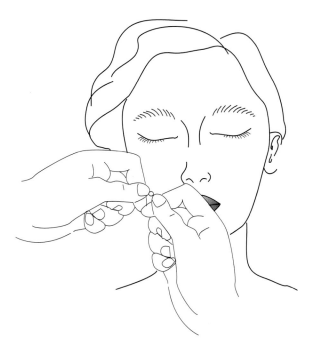

Expressing the contents of a comedone by finger pressure.

- **Closed comedone (whitehead)**: If the comedone does not open easily, it should be punctured gently in its centre with a sterile needle. Following that, the contents of the comedone should be expressed by pressure as described above.

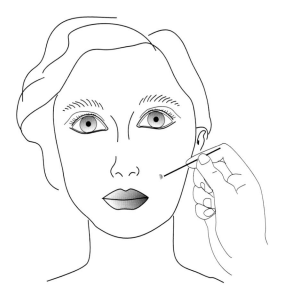

Puncturing a comedone.

- The contents of **small pustules** (up to about 3 mm in diameter) may be drained by puncturing the centre. Following the puncturing, the contents should be expressed with pressure as described above. For the treatment of

larger pustules, the patient should be referred to a doctor. If there are more than four or five pustules, the patient might also be referred to a doctor.

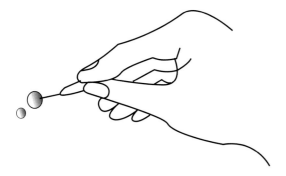

Puncturing a pustule.

- On the other hand, **nodules** or **cysts** should not be punctured or squeezed. These must be treated by a dermatologist.
- **Inflamed, red papules**: One must avoid any manipulation of inflamed lesions. They should not be touched, squeezed or punctured. If punctured, they will just bleed without any drainage of the follicle's content. Fiddling with inflamed papules will only result in unnecessary tissue damage, which can later develop into a scar. No fatty or purulent (pussy) material can be obtained from such a lesion.

Further cleansing
After treatment, it is recommended that the area be cleansed again with alcohol or another antiseptic solution.

Treatment by a dermatologist

In this section, a short summary is presented concerning the treatment of acne by a dermatologist. Two types of treatment are performed by a dermatologist:

- using preparations for external use, applying them to the skin
- using medications given by mouth (systemic treatment)

Note: This section is not presented so as to encourage cosmeticians to treat acne sufferers with medications. Its aim is to broaden cosmeticians' knowledge of the subject, and to let them know which medications are commonly used for acne. Obviously, medicinal treatment may only be given by a physician.

Preparations for external use (application to the skin)
Preparations for external use are designed to be applied to the skin in the areas affected by acne. They are usually in the form of creams or liquids (as emulsions, suspensions, aqueous solutions or alcoholic solutions). These

preparations generally cause drying and scaling of the skin to a variable degree; this is particularly true of those preparations that cause a decrease in the amount of sebum secreted in the skin.

When starting to use a preparation for the first time, one should be cautious: first the substance should be applied over a small area of the skin that is out of sight, and only if no skin irritation occurs can it be applied over a wider affected area and over the face.

It is possible and acceptable practice to use a combination of different preparations: for example, one type of preparation in the morning and a different one for nighttime use.

Preparations containing salicylic acid, sulfur or resorcinol

These are the 'traditional' preparations, which are less commonly used nowadays, since newer preparations have been found to be much more effective. These preparations are **keratolytic** substances – meaning that they dissolve the keratinous substance (keratin) in the skin. Dissolving the keratinous layer helps by enabling removal of the material that is plugging up the opening of the hair follicle. However, the keratolytic action of salicylic acid, sulfur and resorcinol is considered to be weak. These preparations have a drying effect and may irritate the skin. They have mild antibacterial properties.

Alpha-hydroxy acids

The main rationale for using alpha-hydroxy acids in acne is that these preparations, as chemical exfoliants, weaken the adhesion between the degenerating and dead cells of the outer layers of the skin, thereby preventing plugging up of hair follicles. Research has demonstrated the beneficial effect of alpha-hydroxy acids at low concentrations in mild and moderate acne, with subsequent reductions in the number of acne lesions. In low concentrations, they are intended for once- or twice-daily application. Alpha-hydroxy acids are discussed in more detail in Chapter 17.

Benzoyl peroxide

This is an antimicrobial substance that acts by oxidizing the bacterial proteins. When applied to the skin, it penetrates the follicles and decreases the bacterial population of the follicle, which is responsible for the various phenomena of acne. In addition, it has a certain keratolytic effect. It is available in the following forms:

- cream
- gel
- lotion
- facial mask
- in some soaps used for acne

Benzoyl peroxide is usually used in concentrations of 2.5%, 5% or 10%. Preparations containing benzoyl peroxide may cause drying and irritation. Hence it is advisable to begin with a lower concentration, and, if there is no skin irritation, then to move up to a higher concentration.

Antibiotic preparations for external application

These contain one of the following antibiotics:

- erythromycin
- clindamycin
- tetracycline

These preparations act directly on the bacteria in the hair follicle. Their use could potentially result in allergic reactions in a minute percentage of patients.

Retinoic acid

Retinoic acid is chemically related to vitamin A. Its main effect is to regulate the rate of reproduction of cells within the follicle. In that way, it ensures an effective turnover of cells within the follicle, with more effective disposal of dead cells. It thereby prevents the formation of 'plugs' that block the opening of the follicle, thus preventing the formation of comedones. Hence it is particularly useful in non-inflamed acne, which consists mainly of open and closed comedones. Retinoic acid is present in various preparations, which may be in the form of a solution, gel or cream.

The usual concentrations of retinoic acid are 0.025% and 0.05%. When it is first used, the skin may become red and scaly, but after a few weeks of use the irritation subsides. Sometimes, at the beginning of the treatment, there may be a transient worsening of the acne, but this resolves with time. Retinoic acid increases the skin's sensitivity to sunlight; therefore it should be applied only at night. During the day, people using retinoic acid should avoid exposure to sunlight as much as possible, and should apply a sunscreen preparation. Retinoic acid is used to prevent ageing of the skin, and for lightening dark areas of skin as well. There are more details regarding those effects in Chapter 16.

Adapalene

The mechanism of action of adapalene, a drug used for topical treatment in acne, is similar to that of retinoic acid. Adapalene is incorporated in gel preparations, in a concentration of 0.1%. Research has demonstrated the beneficial effect of adapalene in mild to moderate acne. It has some anti-inflammatory activity.

The adverse effects of adapalene basically resemble those of retinoic acid. Skin irritation may occur, manifested by redness, dry skin, and a sensation of stinging, itching or burning.

Adapalene preparations are applied as a thin film on the affected skin areas, once before bedtime, after washing the face.

Azelaic acid

Azelaic acid is produced naturally in the body. Based on this substance, several relatively new preparations have been developed that have been found to be effective, to a certain degree, against acne. Azelaic acid has a combined therapeutic activity: it is both antibacterial and anti-inflammatory. In addition, azelaic acid regulates the cell turnover within the follicle, and in that way prevents blockage of the follicle by keratinous material, and hence the formation of comedones. Preparations containing azelaic acid are useful for both inflammatory and non-inflammatory acne lesions.

Azelaic acid is also used in lightening dark, pigmented areas of skin (see Chapter 18 on bleaching).

Orally administered medications (systemic treatment)

Antibiotics

Antibiotics are used in acne for inflamed and infected lesions. They are direct-ed against the bacteria in the follicle that result in inflammatory acne lesions. The antibiotics generally used in acne are:

- tetracyclines
- erythromycin

Of the antibiotics that can be taken orally, tetracyclines are usually preferred. The most popular medication of this group is **minocycline**. It is given in a dosage of 50 mg twice daily for several weeks. Following that, the patient con-tinues on a maintenance dose of one 50 mg tablet a day for a variable period. The main effect of minocycline is against those bacteria that are involved in the development of acne; however, it has a general effect against inflammato-ry processes as well. (**Doxycycline** is another medication of the tetracycline group that is commonly used in acne.)

Tetracyclines

Since tetracyclines are common medications in the treatment of acne, it is impor-tant to note the following:

- While taking tetracyclines, exposure to sunlight should be minimized, since these drugs increase the skin's sensitivity to sunlight. People who are exposed to sunlight while taking tetracyclines may develop an exaggerated sunburn.
- Drinking milk or eating milk products, such as cheese, together with tetracy-clines interferes with the absorption of the medication in the body, lessening its effect. At least two hours should elapse between taking a tetracycline and ingesting a milk product. Similarly, tetracyclines should not be taken together with antacid preparations, substances containing iron or preparations contain-ing vitamins.
- Tetracyclines can affect the efficacy of contraceptive pills. Therefore women taking the Pill should consult their physicians regarding the use of additional or alternative contraceptive precautions while taking tetracyclines.
- **Tetracyclines must not be taken during pregnancy!**
- Tetracyclines should not be given to children under the age of 14. (In special cases, doctors may consider prescribing medication to younger children.)

Hormonal preparations

The commonly accepted hormonal preparations in the treatment of acne contain an oestrogen (ethinyloestradiol) and/or an anti-androgenic substance that counteracts the male hormones (cyproterone acetate). These preparations are usually used as birth control pills, prescribed by a gynaecologist. Sometimes they are also used for the prevention of excessive hair growth in women.

Isotretinoin

Isotretinoin is an orally administered medication from the retinoid group of compounds – substances that are chemically similar to vitamin A. It is widely known as **Accutane**. The use of isotretinoin results in the following:

- reduction in size of sebaceous glands;
- decrease in activity of sebaceous glands, thus decreasing sebum excretion;
- reduction of the bacterial population within the follicles;
- an anti-inflammatory action, reducing the level of inflammation in follicles;
- restoration of the keratin formation process and the return of cells (turnover) within the follicle to a normal state.

This is an efficacious drug that has been found to be highly beneficial in the treatment of acne that has not responded to previous modalities. In the medical literature, success rates of isotretinoin are reported to be approximately 85–90%. In most patients treated according to the accepted medical guidelines, acne will not appear again. In a few cases when it does, it tends to appear in a mild form.

What are the side-effects of isotretinoin?

- Dryness of the skin appears during the first few weeks of treatment. The skin may peel and become scaly.
- There is increased skin sensitivity to sunlight. This sensitivity can range from mild redness on the face to severe rashes, following excessive exposure to the sun.
- There may be dryness in the mouth, with possible bleeding from the nose (as a result of the dryness). Lip irritation with scaling may occur.
- Hair loss (transient) may occur.
- Disturbance of liver function (usually transient) is possible. Liver function should be monitored in patients receiving isotretinoin, by periodic blood tests, at least once a month.

There may be other side-effects; those listed above are the most common.

The usual course of side-effects when taking isotretinoin

Usually in the first or second week, there is dryness of the skin and mucous membranes (inside the mouth and nose). In the second week of treatment, there may actually be a mild worsening of the acne. However, in the third week of treatment, the inflammatory acne lesions lessen, and from the fourth week onwards, there is gradual healing of most of the acne lesions.

Note:

- **It is not recommended that isotretinoin be given before puberty**.
- **Isotretinoin must not be taken during pregnancy!** If taken during pregnancy, it may cause fetal malformations, particularly in the heart and nervous system. The patient must not become pregnant for at least one month after discontinuation of isotretinoin. In any case, this medication is only ever taken after consulting a physician and a medical examination; it requires a doctor's prescription and monthly follow-up.

Adjusting treatment to the nature and course of acne

Treatment is adjusted to the clinical appearance of the acne.

Mild acne

In mild acne, the aim is to rely on externally applied preparations, that is preparations to be applied locally to the affected areas of skin. If the only lesions are comedones, preparations containing salicylic acid, sulfur or resorcinol usually suffice; alternatively, one can use preparations containing retinoic acid, alpha-hydroxy acids or azaleic acid. In acne, where there are **inflammatory lesions** (such as papules or pustules), one adds antibacterial treatment: benzoyl peroxide or antibiotics applied to the skin (such as erythromycin or clindamycin solutions). A combination of preparations can be used, such as one type in the morning and a different type at night.

Severe acne

Here orally administered medications are usually necessary in addition to local treatment. The treatment is usually based on antibiotics (generally tetracyclines), special contraceptive pills for females, or isotretinoin.

Final comment

Both the physician and the cosmetician must make it clear to the patient that the standard medical treatment of acne is very effective. Over 90% of acne sufferers will show significant improvement within months. Even patients who do not see any improvement within a few months should not despair. There is an extremely wide range of possibilities available for acne treatment, and it is more than likely that one of these treatments will help the patient.

10

Sun and the skin

Contents Overview • Solar radiation; ultraviolet radiation • Short-term effects of sun exposure • Long-term effects of sun exposure: solar damage • Types of skin • Protection from the sun • Addenda: artificial tanning and alteration of skin colour

Overview

There has been increasing awareness of the damage caused to skin by cumulative sun exposure. Solar radiation is responsible for most of the deleterious skin conditions that are sometime erroneously attributed to ageing, such as:

- the appearance of 'sun spots' – those brown spots that tend to appear on areas of skin exposed to the sun;
- the appearance and accentuation of wrinkles and 'sagging' skin;
- enlargement of blood capillaries on the face;
- development of various skin tumours.

This chapter discusses the effects of exposure to the sun – both short-term and long-term effects. The main line of defence against sun exposure is avoidance. In order to protect the skin, one can use sunscreens, also discussed in this chapter.

Solar radiation; ultraviolet radiation

The sun's radiation ranges over a wide spectrum of wavelengths. Visible light, made up of the familiar colours of the rainbow, is in fact only a thin band of the wide total range of radiation, as shown in the illustration on the next page.

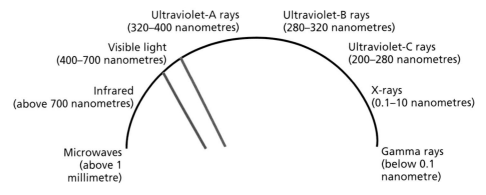

Ultraviolet-A rays
(320–400 nanometres)

Ultraviolet-B rays
(280–320 nanometres)

Visible light
(400–700 nanometres)

Ultraviolet-C rays
(200–280 nanometres)

Infrared
(above 700 nanometres)

X-rays
(0.1–10 nanometres)

Microwaves
(above 1
millimetre)

Gamma rays
(below 0.1
nanometre)

The wide spectrum of wavelengths of the sun's electromagnetic radiation.

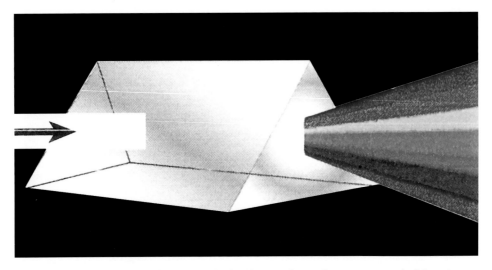

*A glass prism can split **visible light** into the familiar rainbow colours. At one end of the rainbow, the light is red, with a wavelength of about 700 nanometres. At the other end of the rainbow is violet light, with a wavelength of about 400 nanometres. In between lie the other colours of the rainbow. It should be remembered, though, that visible light is only a narrow band that makes up a small fraction of all radiation emanating from the sun. In the spectrum of electromagnetic radiation, those light rays whose wavelengths go beyond those of the visible violet light are called **ultraviolet rays.***

The wavelength of ultraviolet radiation is adjacent to that of visible violet light. Ultraviolet-B (UVB) rays are high-energy emissions, which can cause significant damage to living tissues and cells. This is the main type of radiation that is responsible for:

- reddening and skin burns following exposure to the sun
- tanning

- the appearance of skin tumours following prolonged, cumulative exposure to the sun

The energy level of ultraviolet-A (UVA) rays is less than that of UVB rays, so they cause less skin damage. Until recently, UVA rays were thought to provide 'safe tanning', and most tanning parlours still use lamps that emit UVA for achieving a tan. However, even UVA rays cause skin damage. Moreover, UVA rays penetrate deeper into the skin than do UVB rays, causing damage to the elastin fibres locate deeper in the skin, and thus hastening skin ageing.

Another fact that must be kept in mind is that UVB rays do not penetrate glass, while UVA rays do. Therefore, for example, when driving in a car with closed windows, skin damage can occur because of the UVA radiation. Hence, in an air-conditioned car, one tends to forget that the skin is still exposed to ultraviolet radiation. Therefore:

- It is not advisable to expose oneself to the sun – even through a glass window.
- Treatment at a tanning parlour may damage skin.

Short-term effects of sun exposure

What is suntanning?
When we talk of 'suntanning', we mean that the skin colour darkens. From a medical point of view, suntanning is, in fact the natural mechanism by which the skin protects itself: the sun's rays that reach the epidermis cause the **melanocytes** – special cells in the epidermis – to produce **melanin**, which is the

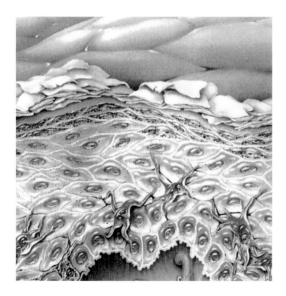

Melanocytes – the melanin-producing cells – at the base of the epidermis.

coloured compound (pigment) that makes the skin darker. Melanin provides the skin with natural protection against solar damage. However, the amount of melanin that is produced in fair-skinned people following exposure to the sun is relatively low and does not afford them adequate protection, and they must take additional precautions against solar skin damage. In dark-skinned people, the amount of melanin produced is higher, and is consequently more effective. That is why dark-skinned people often look younger than fair-skinned people of the same age: in the former, the skin changes less with age, and wrinkles and pigmented patches appear less frequently. Nevertheless, even dark-skinned people should avoid excessive sun exposure. In every case, the less the exposure, the less the damage.

Summary

Tanning is the skin's defence against solar radiation. A tan is the result of the production of melanin as a result of exposure to ultraviolet rays. Tanning does afford the skin a certain degree of protection – but usually not sufficient to prevent solar damage. Prolonged exposure will, over the years, result in the appearance of pigmented patches, abnormal skin texture, wrinkles and sagging of the skin. Later, skin tumours may appear.

Redness and burns following sun exposure

Apart from tanning, ultraviolet radiation also causes redness. The medical term for this redness is **erythema** – and its appearance following exposure to the sun has nothing to do with melanin production. Erythema begins soon after exposure to ultraviolet light – some 4 hours following exposure – reaching its peak 24 hours thereafter. Excessive exposure can cause significant reddening, to the extent of actual skin burns. A mild burn (termed **first-degree**) is manifested by redness with pain and sensitivity of the skin. A deeper burn (**second-degree**) appears following more prolonged exposure to the sun, and is manifested by the appearance of blisters, peeling and severe pain. The treatment of first-degree burns is based on cooling the burnt area by rinsing with water. 'Soothing' applications can also be used, such as those containing aloe vera. A second-degree burn (or a relatively severe or widespread first-degree burn) requires medical attention. In second-degree burns, **antibacterial preparations** (which inhibit or kill bacteria and prevent infection of the burn) may be used. Silver sulfadiazine, an effective product for treating burns, is active against bacteria, and cools and soothes the burnt area. It may be used in cases of severe sunburn.

Two additional comments

- Cumulative damage to the skin as a result of sun exposure can occur following many individual periods of exposure, each of which in itself is not sufficient to cause the skin to become red. Obviously, if a burn does actually occur, the damage is much more serious.
- Evidence has been accumulating that there may be a direct connection between the appearance of **melanoma** – a malignant skin cancer – and excessive exposure to the sun in childhood. Episodes of excessive exposure

to the sun that were associated with severe skin burns may contribute to the development of melanoma appearing many years later.

Other immediate complications of excessive exposure to the sun
Other short-term risks of sun exposure are:

- dehydration
- heatstroke (sunstroke)

Although we draw attention to these risks, these problems are not detailed in this chapter.

Vitamin D and the sun
Vitamin D is needed by the body to build and strengthen bones. Exposure to sunlight stimulates the production of vitamin D in humans. It should be noted, however, that the amount of sunlight needed to produce the vitamin D required by the body is minimal: exposing a few square centimetres of skin for a few minutes daily is sufficient. There is a reasonable amount of vitamin D in most people's diet, even without taking any special steps to ensure it. It must be obvious from all of the above that worrying about an adequate supply of vitamin D is certainly no justification for excessive sun exposure.

Long-term effects of sun exposure: solar damage

Cumulative solar radiation is a direct cause of skin damage. The changes that occur as a result of exposure to the sun are not the same as those processes that occur with natural ageing of the skin. The former are known technically as **photoageing**, and occur in all skin layers – both the epidermis and the dermis.

Remember that exposure to the sun occurs not only at the beach or on hikes. In most people, certain parts of the body, particularly the face, neck, and backs of the hands, are exposed to the sun for more than an hour a day, and sometimes even more. We are talking of daily exposure over years, and it is clear that such cumulative exposure has significant effects on the health of the skin.

Effects on the epidermis
Cumulative solar exposure leads to the appearance of wrinkles, and an uneven distribution of pigment in the skin. This is caused by the exposure of melanocytes (the pigment-producing cells) in the epidermis to the sun. In young people, prolonged solar exposure may express itself in the form of freckles. In older people, the solar exposure leads to the appearance of **'sun spots'** (**solar lentigines**), which are brown blotches on the skin. In everyday language, these patches are often called 'age spots' or 'liver spots'. One can see these lesions in older people in those areas usually exposed to the sun, such as the face and the backs of the hands.

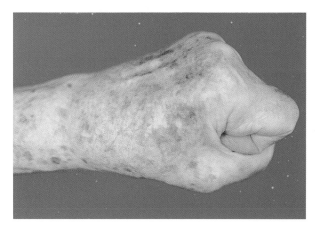

'Sun spots' (solar lentigines) on the back and side of the hand.

Other solar damage as a result of cumulative exposure to the sun includes the appearance of skin tumours – both benign and malignant (see Chapter 14 on skin tumours). Common tumours that result from cumulative solar exposure are:

- solar keratosis
- basal cell carcinoma
- squamous cell carcinoma

It is important to prevent excessive exposure to the sun in children. Current thinking is that the appearance of **malignant melanoma**, a particularly dangerous malignant skin cancer, is related to episodes of excessive exposure to the sun in childhood. It should be noted that in this particular case, we are not talking of cumulative exposure to the sun, but of episodes of excessive exposure resulting in a severe sunburn.

Effects on the dermis
The changes in the dermis are as follows:

- The main damage to the dermis following cumulative exposure to the sun is the destruction of elastin and collagen fibres; these fibres confer upon the skin its elasticity and strength. If they are damaged, the skin loses its elasticity, becomes wrinkled, and appears 'saggy'.
- In addition, cumulative exposure to the sun damages the delicate blood vessels of the skin and the supporting tissues. The blood vessels become more fragile, and in that situation haemorrhages (bleeding) can occur in the skin following relatively minor injury.
- Similarly, the capillary blood vessels of the face may enlarge – a phenomenon known as **telangiectasis**.
- Excessive exposure to the sun makes the skin dry. When there is constant dryness of the skin over a prolonged period of time, the skin's health and quality is affected.

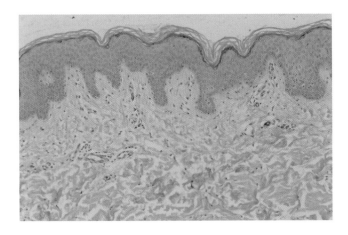

Healthy skin viewed through a microscope.

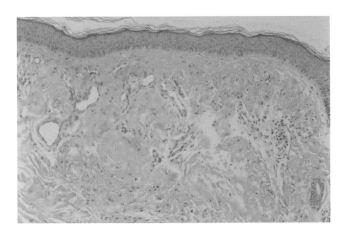

Photodamaged skin viewed through a microscope, showing thinning of the epidermis following long exposure to the sun.

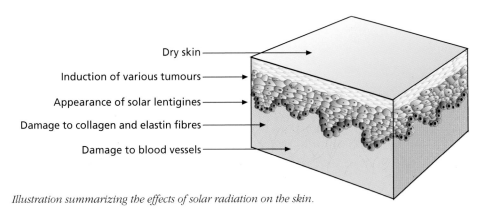

Dry skin

Induction of various tumours

Appearance of solar lentigines

Damage to collagen and elastin fibres

Damage to blood vessels

Illustration summarizing the effects of solar radiation on the skin.

The above description explains why, in older people with fair complexions, the skin in those areas exposed to the sun (face, neck, upper chest), looks 'old' and wrinkled, while the skin that is not exposed to the sun (buttocks, abdomen and inner part of the arms) looks smooth, clear and younger.

Note: Exposing the eyes to strong radiation, without adequate protection, can cause damage to the lens of the eye, with the risk of developing a cataract. There is also evidence suggesting that cumulative exposure to solar radiation may also damage the retina of the eye.

Types of skin

The classification of skin into different types is based on the skin colour, its propensity for developing sunburn, its tanning capability and the degree of tanning. The parameters measured are the propensity for getting burned after 30 minutes of exposure to the sun at noon in early summer. Depending on these factors, one can determine the degree of protection needed against solar radiation.

Skin type 1
People with type 1 skin have pale skin, commonly have blond or red hair, and have light-coloured eyes. If these people are exposed to bright sun for 30 minutes, they will always get sunburn. They never tan.

Skin type 2
Most of these people have a fair complexion and light-coloured eyes. If a person with type 2 skin stays in the sun for about 30 minutes, his/her skin will usually develop redness and sunburn. Some of these people tan, but only after repeated sun exposures.

Skin type 3
In this group, there is a wide spectrum of skin complexions, ranging from relatively fair to relatively darker shades. All those with type 3 skin can develop a suntan, although the length of time needed to develop a deep tan is variable. After sun exposure of 30 minutes, they will tan, although the degree of tanning varies from one person to another. Following prolonged sun exposure, they may sunburn.

Skin type 4
People in this group generally have dark hair, brown or black eyes, and a relatively dark complexion. Most of the population of North Africa are in this category. They develop an even tan after 30 minutes of exposure to the sun (but will not burn after 30 minutes of sun exposure).

Skin type 5
This group comprises dark-skinned people (e.g. people from India). They rarely sunburn, and always tan readily.

Skin type 6
People in this group (e.g. people of African origin) have skin that is dark even in areas never exposed to the sun. When exposed to the sun, their skin darkens to a deep brown/black shade. They do not sunburn.

Note: In order to identify types 5 and 6, there is no need to test the skin after 30 minutes of sun exposure – it is sufficient to observe the skin colour.

Protection from the sun

Protection is essentially based on avoidance of exposure. We emphasize that the same rays that cause tanning are the ones that cause damage. The lighter the person's skin, the more susceptible it is to solar damage. The purpose of a sunscreen is not to help tanning, but rather to block the sun's rays. In other words, ideally one should not be exposed to the sun. However, if someone is going to be exposed to the sun anyhow (at the beach, on a hike or at work), he/she should at least make sure that his/her skin is protected by a sunscreen and appropriate clothing.

The typical advertisements for sunscreens generally show a suntanned model smearing a sunscreen preparation all over herself, then basking in the hot sun. That message is misleading:

- The belief that sunscreens help achieve a suntan is not correct.
- The belief that sunscreens filter out only the 'harmful' rays is not correct.
- Harmful ultraviolet rays may definitely pass through sunscreens.

We stress that it is preferable to avoid exposure to the sun. However, if for any reason someone has to be in open area exposed to the sun then he/she should apply a sunscreen. Of the multi-billion dollar 'beauty' market, and of all the products that promise to keep the face 'young', there is nothing that comes anywhere near the simple act of avoiding exposure to the sun.

How to avoid exposure to the sun

- The times of outdoor activities should be planned for those hours when the level of solar radiation is relatively low. Exposure to the sun should be avoided as much as possible between the hours of 9 am and 4 pm, which is when the sun's radiation is strongest.
- During outdoor activities, it is important to keep to the shade as much as possible, and to wear appropriate clothing. It should be remembered that a large amount of solar radiation is reflected from water, sand and concrete pavements – all of which a person may be exposed to even when sitting in the shade. A beach umbrella does not guarantee complete protection from the sun: ultraviolet rays are reflected from all sorts of reflective surfaces, so that even under a beach umbrella one needs protection by wearing suitable clothing or a sunscreen preparation. For the same reason, a hat does not afford full protection against the sun.
- Cloudy days tend to be cooler and with relatively less sunshine, but a considerable percentage of the ultraviolet rays penetrate clouds, and even on cloudy days – especially relatively bright days – appropriate protective measures must be taken.

- Severe sunburn can occur in snow, because of reflection of a relatively high percentage of the sun's rays from the snow. Furthermore, the higher the altitude, the more solar radiation gets through to the earth, since the rays have to travel through a thinner layer of atmosphere (which filters the rays to some extent). Hence, when in an area of snow, it is important to protect the exposed areas, particularly the face and ears.
- Most clothing protects effectively against the sun's rays, because it either absorbs or reflects the ultraviolet rays. In general, the thicker the material, and the tighter the weave, the higher the level of protection it affords. The colour of the material is also a factor: different colours absorb or reflect rays to different degrees, and the protective capabilities of a material are related to the chemical composition of the various dyes. Dyeing a cloth may raise its sun protection factor (SPF – see below) by 4 or more, compared with white cloth.

  White material allows quite a lot of ultraviolet radiation to pass through it, so that someone who wears a thin white T-shirt may still absorb about 20% as much radiation as if he had a bare torso. Wearing a thin shirt of that kind is approximately equivalent to using a sunscreen with an SPF of between 4 and 10, depending on the thickness, density of weave and type of material of the shirt. Material such as that is not always sufficient protection against solar radiation. Furthermore, if the shirt is wet, its protective capability decreases by 30–40% compared with when it is dry.

  In addition, wearing tight clothes decreases the protective effects of the material, because stretching the material opens up the spaces between its threads in the weave. Thick woollen clothing, denim and clothes made of polyester fibres afford good protection against solar radiation.

Sunscreens

Physical and chemical sunscreens

Until the 1970s, the attitude towards tanning preparations was that they were essentially cosmetic preparations designed to increase tanning and prevent sunburn. Since the late 1970s, the importance of sunscreens in protecting the skin from solar damage has been more strongly emphasized.

Sunscreens may be physical or chemical. Most sunscreen preparations contain both physical and chemical sunscreens, and may be in the form of a cream, an ointment, an emulsion, a gel, etc.

Physical sunscreens prevent the sun's rays from reaching the skin by reflecting and dispersing them, as a mirror reflects light rays. The major component of physical sunscreens is a substance similar to talc called **titanium dioxide**.

Chemical sunscreens absorb ultraviolet rays, and in that way prevent them from penetrating the skin. The degree of absorption depends on the particular substance used, and its concentration. Substances used as chemical sunscreens are **oxybenzone**, **benzophenones** and **para-aminobenzoic acid** (**PABA**). These names can be found on the packages of different sunscreen preparations.

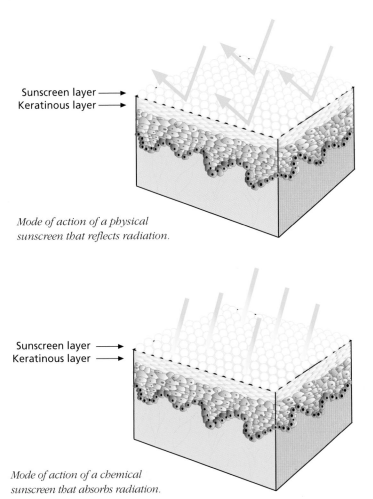

Sunscreen layer ⟶
Keratinous layer ⟶

Mode of action of a physical sunscreen that reflects radiation.

Sunscreen layer ⟶
Keratinous layer ⟶

Mode of action of a chemical sunscreen that absorbs radiation.

Blocking ultraviolet rays with sunscreens
Most chemical sunscreens block 95% of the UVB rays; most do not block UVA rays. Chemical sunscreens of the benzophenone group, as well as the physical sunscreens, block ultraviolet rays more completely, provided their sun protection factor is above 15. In general, an ideal combination is a physical sunscreen combined with a chemical sunscreen.

What does 'sun protection factor' mean?
The term **sun protection factor** (**SPF**) was adopted by the US Food and Drug Administration (FDA). This measurement allows one to assess the degree of protection from ultraviolet rays provided to the skin by a sunscreen, compared with the skin without sunscreen.

The effectiveness of a given SPF is measured in terms of the redness that appears on the skin following sun exposure. This redness is known medically as **erythema**. The concept of a **minimal erythema dose** is an expression of the minimal amount of radiation that causes reddening of the skin. This radiation dose varies from person to person, depending on his/her skin shade and type. For example, if it takes someone without any sunscreen 10 minutes of sun exposure to develop erythema, exposure to that same strength of sunlight using a sunscreen with an SPF of 15 will take 150 minutes (10 × 15) to develop erythema.

Characteristics of various sunscreens

The preparation's endurance on the skin: According to the FDA's definitions:

- A **water-resistant** product provides skin protection even after 40 minutes of immersion in (fresh) water.
- A **waterproof** product retains its protective capabilities after 80 minutes of immersion in (fresh) water.
- A product that does not lose more than 25% of its effectiveness after a 40 minute swim is recognized as water-resistant.
- A product that loses over 25% of its effectiveness after a 40 minute swim is *not* water-resistant. One must apply sunscreens repeatedly to exposed skin during sun exposure.

Skin sensitivity: This tends to be more of a problem with chemical sunscreens. In the past, para-aminobenzoic acid was used in most sunscreens, but in recent years the trend has been to replace it with other sunscreens of the oxybenzone and benzophenone groups, which cause less skin irritation. Physical sunscreens, on the other hand, generally do not cause skin reactions. In many cases, skin sensitivity from contact with sunscreens is caused by other ingredients in the preparation, such as the perfumes or preservatives, and not necessarily by the sunscreen itself.

Stinging of the eyes: This is a common side-effect experienced after applying a sunscreen. The stinging sensation is most commonly related to irritation of the eyes from the fumes of the preparation. People who encounter this problem should change to a different sunscreen (preferably a physical sunscreen that contains titanium dioxide). In general, any sunscreen can cause irritation if it comes into direct contact with the eyes, as a result of the user rubbing the eyes after applying the preparation, or because the sunscreen is too 'runny'. Water-resistant sunscreens tend to be less 'runny', and are recommended for the area around the eyes.

Important properties of a sunscreen and which sunscreens should be preferred?

Sun protection factor (SPF): Ideally this should be 15 or greater. For people with skin type 1 or 2, and for certain people at high risk (such as those with an increased risk of skin tumours), SPF 30 or greater is necessary. The recommended SPF depends not only on the person's skin type, but also on the length of time he/she intends to spend in the sun.

Note: A sunscreen is considered to afford effective protection only if it has an SPF of 15 or greater. A sunscreen with SPF 15 blocks about 93% of UVB radiation. A sunscreen with SPF 30 blocks about 97% of UVB radiation. In sunscreens with SPF higher than 30, the additional improvement in the protection from ultraviolet radiation is minimal: increasing the SPF from 30 to 40 increases UVB protection by less than 1%.

How long does the product stay on the skin? One must know how long the sunscreen preparation will stay on the skin after applying it, and how often one has to apply it again. Its resistance to water and sweat should also be assessed.

Characteristics such as the product's colour or texture; the feeling it leaves on the skin: If a sunscreen leaves one with an unpleasant feeling on the face, presumably one can find an alternative and more satisfactory product with the same SPF.

Does the product irritate the skin or eyes? If the sunscreen does cause irritation, one should try another one.

How to use a sunscreen

The preparation should be applied to all exposed areas of skin, in particular the face, ears, neck, upper chest, backs of the hands, and bald areas of the head in males. It should be noted that sunscreen preparations dissolve in sweat, and, like other creams, come off following immersion in water or with rubbing. A water-resistant sunscreen should be re-applied every three to four hours; a sunscreen that is less water-resistant should be re-applied even more frequently. Every sunscreen should be re-applied after immersion in water, swimming, etc. During physical exercise, sport, etc., that causes sweating that removes the sunscreen, it should be applied more frequently. The sunscreen should ideally be applied some 30 minutes before going out into the sun, so that it has time to penetrate into the keratinous layer of the skin. However, if that is not done, it should be applied every time one goes out into the sun.

Note: We repeat that no sunscreen is 100% effective. Someone who stays in the sun for a long time exposes him/herself to solar damage, including possible burns, and skin damage from cumulative exposure to ultraviolet rays.

Final comments regarding sunscreens

Recent studies tend to show a statistical increase in the incidence of skin tumours among the general population, in spite of the increasing awareness and use of sunscreen preparations. The main reason is apparently that these preparations, promoted extensively by advertising, have produced a feeling of complacency. They encourage their users to expose themselves to the sun, by giving a false sense of security and protection, which in fact does not exist. It must be remembered that, by staying in the sun for a lengthy period, even someone who religiously covers him/herself with a sunscreen will allow his/her skin to absorb a certain amount of radiation, which also causes skin damage.

Sunscreens are the last line of defence against the sun. They are designed to offer some protection to those areas of the body, such as the face and hands, that are unavoidably exposed to the sun. The first line of defence is to keep out of the sun as much as possible.

Sunscreen preparations offer some protection to those people who, for whatever reason (occupation or leisure activities) have no alternative but to be in the sun. Under those circumstances, they should use a sunscreen to minimize the damage. Advertisements that show people smearing themselves with a sunscreen preparation so that they can then frolic in the sun, with 'safe, healthy suntanning', are misleading and deceptive.

Another criticism has been levelled against the use of the sun protection factor (SPF) as a measure of the effectiveness of a sunscreen preparation

The SPF of a sunscreen is determined by its ability to prevent the appearance of reddening of the skin (erythema) following exposure to the sun. This means that, by comparing one sunscreen with another in terms of their SPFs, one can tell how much each one delays the appearance of erythema. However, that does not necessarily tell us how effective the sunscreen is in preventing the appearance of malignant tumours on the skin, or its ability to prevent damage to the skin. Studies that have examined the effectiveness of sunscreens in the prevention of these phenomena have showed varying results. In any case, it is also necessary to be strict and to apply sunscreens together with avoiding exposure to the sun.

Additional tips on protection from the sun

Protect the nose
One needs to be particularly careful to protect the nose from the sun and to apply sunscreen more frequently. The nose receives the most exposure to the sun, and is at a particularly high risk of developing solar damage. Furthermore, if skin cancer develops on the nose, the tumour will have to be removed, and it should be noted that:

• Scars on the nose following removal of lesions always look more prominent because of the nose's central position on the face.

• The skin of the nose tends to form relatively thick, unsightly scars.

Protection must be consistent

There is no point in persisting with reasonable protective measures for months, and then one day, at work or at some leisure activity, to be exposed to prolonged radiation and develop a burn. Under such circumstances, the damage will be even worse than usual, because the skin will not have been exposed to the sun previously, and will not have had a chance to develop natural protective means, in the form of production of melanin.

Use sunglasses

Sunglasses protect the eyes as well as the skin. The glasses should be of the type that screen out 100% of ultraviolet rays. It is probably wise to select sunglasses of a reputable, well-known make.

Note: Uncertified plastic sunglasses should never be used. Simple plastic does not filter out ultraviolet light, but in fact blocks the visible light rays, so the damage is even worse! Someone using plastic sunglasses does not constrict his/her pupils in bright light, and an even greater amount of ultraviolet light can get into the eye and cause damage.

Sunglasses also prevent squinting in bright light. Repeated squinting may accelerate the appearance of wrinkles around the eyes, so sunglasses also help to prevent that from occurring. It is preferable to use sunglasses that are elongated and elliptical in shape, similar to the shape of the eye, or glasses with a wider side-bar, to prevent rays reaching the eyes from the sides.

Use a wide-brimmed hat

Hats without a wide brim do not afford effective protection from the sun for the facial skin. Even wide-brimmed hats do not provide effective protection from the sun's rays (they are approximately equivalent to a sunscreen with an SPF of 3). Hence, in any case, even when wearing a wide-brimmed hat, additional protective measures should be taken, such as applying a sunscreen preparation onto the face and avoiding unnecessary exposure to the sun. For bald heads, which are at a high risk of developing solar damage, the hat plays much more significant role in protecting the skin. Bald people should wear hats during outdoor activities.

Protection of the lips

A sunscreen preparation should be used on the lips. Recent research has shown that tumours on the lips are more common in men than in women. The difference was attributed to the widespread use of lipstick by women. The lipstick acts as a filter for the sun's rays, because of the dyes it contains, which function as a physical sunscreen and prevent penetration of the rays to the skin. Tumours of the lips are more common in women who do not use lipstick than in those who use lipstick regularly.

Car windows
A sunshade should be placed inside car windows, since a certain percentage of ultraviolet rays gets through the glass, and may cause cumulative damage (UVA rays certainly penetrate glass). If necessary, special glass can be obtained that filters out most of the ultraviolet rays.

Suntanning and exposure to the sun: how to minimize the damage

For someone who wants to acquire a suntan, in spite of everything that has been said up to this point regarding the damage that exposure to sunlight causes to the skin, we can provide advice to minimize the damage.

- Even when staying in the sun, particular attention should be paid to protecting those areas of skin that are normally exposed in daily activities – the face, backs of the hands, and the nose especially (even in the shade, they absorb ultraviolet rays). A sunscreen preparation should be applied more frequently and generously to those areas. A wide-brimmed hat should be worn to protect the face.
- Exposure to the sun should be avoided in the middle of the day, when the sun is strongest. One should keep out of the sun between 9 am and 4 pm.
- Exposure to the sun should be gradual, so that the skin can gradually build up a protective layer of melanin. Subsequently, once the desired level of tan has been achieved, exposure to the sun should not exceed 30 minutes per day (late in the afternoon), and should not exceed an hour or hour and a half per week – depending on the type of skin. Furthermore, above a certain degree of tanning, increased exposure to the sun will not 'improve' the suntan, but will merely cause skin damage. Having said that, it should be remembered that a suntan does not provide an adequate protective layer to the skin. It may reach a level of protection equivalent to a sunscreen with an SPF of 4–5, depending on the degree of tan and the type of skin.
- Exposure to the sun should be regular, and not just random, whereby each time the skin may absorb excessive amounts of radiation. The damage to the skin is many times worse in someone who is exposed to the sun once for several hours than in someone who is exposed for, say, a quarter of an hour a day once every two or three days, over a period of several weeks (in spite of the fact that in the latter case the total time of exposure to the sun is much longer). The most damage is caused by intermittent, irregular exposure to the sun. Dermatologists consider that the many 'beauty spots' on children's skins are due, apart from hereditary factors, to repeated, irregular exposure to the sun. Furthermore, it is possible that the statistical increase in the incidence of skin cancers in spite of the widespread use of sunscreens is related to irregularity in this use. The classic example of this is the person who is usually very strict and applies sunscreen daily, but forgets to apply it one day when hiking on a sunny day. The damage that is caused in that case may be much worse, since the skin is not protected and not 'ready' for such a huge amount of solar radiation.

People with a skin type that does not tend to tan should minimize sun exposure. Those with skin types 1 or 2 should totally avoid sun exposure.

Possible advantages of sun exposure

In spite of the above, a reasonable amount of controlled exposure to the sun may have certain advantages of which the medical profession may not be fully aware. Thus, for example, being in a well-lit environment (where one is exposed to radiation in the visible range) improves one's mood. This is utilized in psychiatry, in the treatment of depression. Furthermore, some reports (albeit controversial) have appeared in the medical literature suggesting that controlled exposure to the sun may prevent, to some extent, the onset of various malignant diseases.

Addenda: artificial tanning and alteration of skin colour

Artificial tanning ('sunless suntan')

Dihydroxyacetone

Artificial suntanning preparations contain a substance called **dihydroxyacetone** in concentrations of 2.5–10%. The accepted concentration is 5%. This substance reacts with amino acids in the keratin layer of the epidermis, which, it will be recalled, is made up of dead cells. Within a few hours, a suntan-like colour appears in the skin, which may last for three to five days. This colour disappears gradually, as the cells of the outer layers of the epidermis proceed towards the surface of the skin and are shed naturally. Until the outer cells are shed from the skin, the colour resulting from the use of this substance cannot be removed.

Note: Dihydroxyacetone has no medical value. It does not protect the skin from the sun's rays, so an effective sunscreen must be used during exposure to the sun.

The earlier preparations based on dihydroxyacetone were not very effective. However, modern preparations are relatively effective in imparting to the skin a fairly uniform brown toning, which looks reasonably natural – depending on the normal skin colouring.

The following precautions should be adopted when using these preparations:

- Care should be taken to avoid wetting the body for about an hour after applying the preparation, since this would prevent the appearance of the artificial tan.
- The preparation should not be allowed to get onto the scalp hair or the eyebrows, since it may change the colour of the hair.
- The substance should be kept away from clothing, since it may leave stains.

- Before using the preparation, it should be tried out first on a concealed area (that is not normally exposed) to check that there is no adverse reaction, and to confirm that the skin colour is the desired shade (in some people, these preparations result in an unsightly pale-yellowish tinge).
- A thin, even layer of the preparation should be applied – otherwise an uneven, blotchy effect may result, with patches of different shades of colour.
- The hands should be washed after using the preparation to avoid staining the palms.
- A basic soap (i.e. one with a high pH) should not be used to wash the body before applying the preparation, since the resulting colour will tend to be more yellow, rather than the desired brown shade.

Note: If a single application of the preparation does not produce a dark-enough tan, it may be re-applied a few hours later.

Bronzers

These preparations contain a water-soluble pigment (colour) that settles onto the skin. There is no chemical reaction between the pigment and the skin. If the end-result is not what is wanted, the substance can be rinsed off with soap and water. These substances have no effect whatsoever in terms of protection from the sun. The main disadvantage of bronzing agents is that they have to be applied frequently, since they come off every time the skin is washed with soap and water. In summary, these preparations have no medical value. In fact, we are talking of a paint that is applied externally – basically a make-up.

Medications that alter skin colour

These include:

- beta-carotene
- tyrosine
- 'tanning accelerators' – psoralens

Beta-carotene

This substance is chemically similar to vitamin A. It is available as tablets, but is present naturally in large quantities in carrots, tomatoes, mangoes and oranges. When large amounts are ingested, the skin changes colour, becoming an orange-yellow color, and not brown. Nevertheless, if that is combined with exposure to the sun, the additional colour imparted to the skin by the carotene may improve the tanning effect and darken the skin.

> #### Beta-carotene has no effect in terms of protection from ultraviolet rays
>
> However, to some extent, it does block light in the visible spectrum. For most people, this is of no significance. However, certain skin diseases are caused by excessive sensitivity of the skin to sunlight, even within the visible light spectrum. In such cases, beta-carotene is a useful medication for these diseases.

This preparation is available in Europe and Canada as 'tanning pills'; it is not licensed for use in the USA. It should be taken after consultation with a physician, and it is important that a reasonable dosage be taken. If taken in excess (this applies also to people who eat excessive amounts of carrots or mangoes), **hypercarotenemia** may occur, in which the skin goes yellow-orange. If an even higher dosage of 'tanning pills' is taken, it can actually result in poisoning.

Tyrosine
At first glance, there appears to be a certain logic in using tyrosine, since it is the substance from which the pigment melanin is formed. Therefore several preparations containing tyrosine were produced, which were to be applied to the skin prior to exposure to the sun. However, research has not shown any beneficial effect from the use of tyrosine-based preparations.

Psoralens
Psoralens are a group of substances that increase the sensitivity of the skin to ultraviolet radiation, and which cause faster tanning. They are used as medications in skin diseases (such as psoriasis or certain malignant skin diseases), but at the same time that they accelerate tanning, they increase all the deleterious effects on the skin from solar exposure. Hence they are definitely not approved for use as tanning agents.

Tanning parlours
Tanning machines emit ultraviolet irradiation. As stated above, this radiation causes skin damage – both damage that is seen in the skin tissue (the appearance of wrinkles and blotches) and a higher risk of developing skin cancers in later life. There are tanning parlours that claim that their tanning is 'safe', since the machines emit only ultraviolet-A rays. Remember, however, that this radiation also causes damage to the skin. UVA radiation penetrates deeper into the dermis and can damage the elastic tissue of the skin, which will accelerate the appearance of wrinkles. Another problem with tanning parlors is that many people expose their *entire* body to the ultraviolet light, including areas such as around the genitalia, which (one assumes!) have not been exposed to sunlight in the past. Those areas may be at higher risk of developing skin cancer following uncontrolled exposure to ultraviolet light in a tanning parlour.

Tanning oils
These are oils that are applied to the skin. There is a range of oily substances, from various sources – mainly vegetable, such as coconut oil, peanut oil, etc. These substances do not contain any sunscreen agent, and do not protect the skin from the sun. On the contrary, they may actually concentrate the sun's rays on those areas of skin covered with them, and in that way result in even more severe damage.

- They may impede the normal function of sweat glands and sebaceous glands, which could result in the appearance or aggravation of various rashes, for example a rash called **miliaria** ('**prickly heat**'). It may result in a rash of **acne**, manifested mainly by the appearance of comedones.

- The manufacturers' claim that these oils contain vitamins and various natural ingredients that 'nourish' the skin; the beneficial effect on the skin is doubtful (see Chapter 15 on active ingredients in cosmetic preparations).
- The skin colour achieved using these oils is no different from the normal colour that follows exposure to the sun, without any additional substance being applied to the skin.

11

Network of blood vessels on the skin

Contents   Overview • A network of blood vessels on the face is a manifestation of cumulative skin damage • Treatment of telangiectasia on the face • Network of blood vessels on the legs • 'Spider' telangiectasia

Overview

The appearance of a network of fine blood vessels on the skin is common. Cosmeticians sometimes call this **couperose**, although the more widely used medical term for this condition is **telangiectasia**, which refers to dilatation of fine, superficial blood vessels on the surface of the skin. These lesions are known as **telangiectases** (plural of **telangiectasis**).

This chapter discusses:

1 the common appearance of telangiectasia on the face as a manifestation of cumulative damage to the skin;
2 appropriate treatment;
3 appearance of telangiectasia on the legs;
4 other forms of telangiectasia.

A network of blood vessels on the face is a manifestation of cumulative skin damage

Telangiectasia is a common phenomenon, and is the result of cumulative damage to the skin of the face, leading to weakening of the walls of the blood vessels in the skin, and loss of the supporting tissue around the blood vessels.

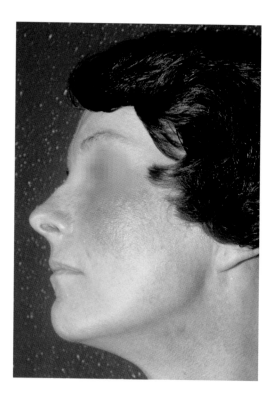

Telangiectasia on the face.

What causes cumulative skin damage, and the subsequent onset of telangiectasia?
This can occur for the following reasons:

- ageing of the skin because of cumulative exposure to the sun;
- exposure to irradiation (in patients with malignant disease);
- following mechanical trauma;
- prolonged application of 'steroid'-containing products to the skin;
- under certain circumstances, telangiectasia appears because of prolonged dilatation of the blood vessels of the face, for example in alcoholism or in certain skin diseases (such as a condition known as **rosacea**).

Telangiectasia that results from cumulative skin damage is usually in the form of lines. The lesions range in colour from pink to dark red, and the diameter of the blood vessels is 0.1–1 mm.

Treatment of telangiectasia on the face

The basic treatment of telangiectasia is aimed at the cause and its prevention. If the underlying cause is alcohol consumption then restricting alcohol improves the situation. If the underlying cause is rosacea, appropriate treatment of this

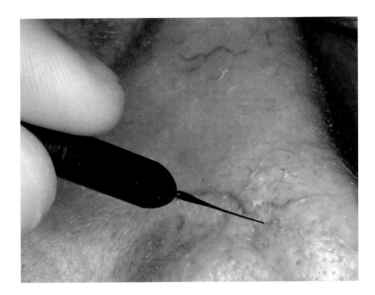

Treating blood vessels with an electric needle.

disease by a dermatologist is required. In any case, exposure to the sun should be minimized, as should exposure to other environmental conditions that may be deleterious to the skin, such as cold or wind.

The dermatologist has several treatment modalities:

Electric cautery with a needle
This is an old method of treatment – it is not sufficiently selective, and may damage tissues around the blood vessels.

Laser treatment
The currently popular treatment is cautery of the telangiectases with a **laser beam**. A laser instrument is used that emits a ray with a wavelength that is precisely matched to the red colour of the blood vessels. If a non-selective laser instrument is used, it may cause unwanted and excessive damage to the tissues around the blood vessels. For more details about this technique, refer to Chapter 23 on laser treatment in dermatology.

Other treatments
Other modern instruments also work on the basis of **brief pulses of light rays** that are not laser rays (for example the ESC 'Photoderm' instrument), and which also are selective for blood vessels. The doctor selects the wavelength appropriate for the colour and the size of the blood vessels being treated.

The blood vessels that form telangiectases on the face are usually superficial (close to the surface), so that **skin peeling** (see Chapter 22) may solve the problem in some cases.

Make-up

Those who do not wish to undergo the above treatments may find that make-up to 'hide' the lesions may be adequate (see Chapter 24 on camouflaging skin lesions).

Network of blood vessels on the legs

Telangiectasia on the legs is related mainly to the problem of hydrostatic pressure, and is the result of poor function of the valves in the leg veins (the medical term for this problem is **venous insufficiency**). Because the valves in the veins do not function adequately, blood tends to pool in the lower part of the leg, and the veins become permanently distended with blood. At first, these veins appear as reddish lines in the skin, which turn blue with time.

Telangiectasia of this nature is common in women over the age of 30, and it tends to appear during pregnancy, so there is reason to believe it is in some way related to hormonal influences.

As mentioned above, telangiectases tend to appear as red or blue lines, sometimes in a lace-like pattern.

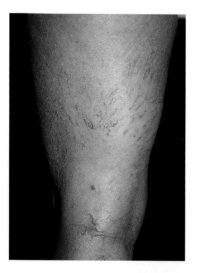

Arborizing telangiectasia.

(a)

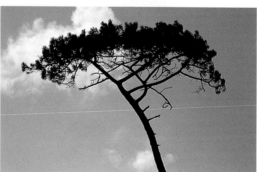

Maritime pine, a natural example of telangiectatic venous drainage and 'feeding' vein.

(b)

There is another form of telangiectasia, which looks like the branches of a tree (**arborizing telangiectasia**); this usually occurs on the outer part of the thighs.

Later in this chapter, we shall deal in more detail with venous insufficiency and its treatment.

Other forms of networks of blood vessels on the skin

Note that in certain cases, telangiectasia can occur as a consequence of certain diseases that affect the connective tissue and blood vessels. These include, for example, diseases such as **lupus**, **scleroderma** and **dermatomyositis**. In general, there is a long list of diseases – some genetically transmitted and some not – that can cause telangiectasia. In rare cases, the appearance of a network of blood vessels on the skin in children is a manifestation of a congenital syndrome. This topic is mentioned here to make the point that telangiectasia under those circumstances is not a cosmetic problem, and the patient should be referred to a dermatologist for diagnosis and treatment.

'Spider' telangiectasia

Another form of telangiectasia is **'spider' telangiectasia**. These lesions tend to occur mainly on the upper half of the body – face, neck and arms. They are usually about 1–1.5 cm in size. Tiny blood vessels radiate from a central artery, as shown in the sketch. If you press exactly on the centre of the lesion with a pencil or penpoint, you can see how the entire lesion 'disappears'. If you then release the pressure from the central artery, the blood vessels all then 'reappear' (in fact, they now fill up with blood and become visible). If you

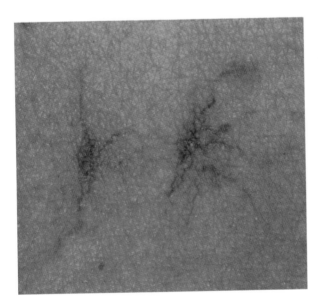

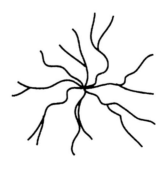

'Spider' telangiectasia.

press lightly with a glass slide on the central artery, you can see pulsation of the artery corresponding to the patient's heart beat.

'Spider' telangiectases normally appear in about 10–20% of the population, and can also be seen normally in children. They occur particularly in women, and are considered to be related to high levels of oestrogen hormones, so they tend to appear under those circumstances when there are high levels of oestrogen – for example in pregnancy, or in patients with certain liver diseases. With regard to pregnancy, more than 50% of pregnant women may develop spider telangiectases. The lesions tend to grow during the pregnancy, and usually disappear within a few weeks after delivery.

In terms of the aesthetic management, these lesions are treated in the same way as other telangiectases.

Venous insufficiency in the legs: an overview

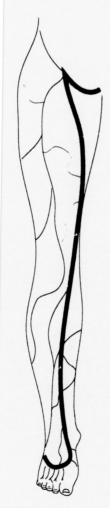

Venous insufficiency in the legs, i.e. inefficient blood flow in the leg veins, leads to varicose veins – relatively large, dilated blood vessels in the lower limbs – as well as to a network of fine blood vessels (telangiectases).

The blood drains from the legs via the veins. There is a system of valves in the veins that ensures that this blood flow is in one direction only (from the feet toward the heart).

The problem is more common in women. With age, there tends to be a weakening and decrease in efficiency of the venous drainage system. That leads to a tendency to dilatation (widening) of the veins. In larger blood vessels, this dilatation results in varicose veins. Since many small veins drain into the larger veins, there is also a 'banking up' of blood in the smaller vessels, which also become dilated, and appear as telangiectases.

The reasons for abnormal blood flow in the legs are partly hereditary and partly hormonal (including the effects of pregnancy). The problem can also appear following inflammation of the veins.

Venous insufficiency leads to swelling of the legs, pain when standing for long periods, and dilatation of superficial veins on the surface of the skin. With more severe venous insufficiency, particularly in old age, the skin around the problem areas may become inflamed. This is a condition known as **stasis dermatitis**, in which the skin appears thicker, becomes dark, and tends to itch.

Blood flow along the leg veins.

What can be done to alleviate venous insufficiency?

- The problem is more severe in people who stand up for long periods of time, so, as far as possible, one should avoid standing for prolonged periods. Furthermore, when sitting, one should not sit with the legs dangling down – rather the legs should rest on a stool or chair (ideally, the feet should be at the height of the buttocks).
- Walking is beneficial, since activating the muscles of the legs helps propel the blood upwards.
- When necessary, elastic stockings may be helpful.
- Each case of problem veins in the legs must be treated on its own merits, following medical consultation.
- If the problem is one of fine telangiectases on the legs, the treatment is the same as for telangiectases elsewhere on the body, and includes cautery with an electric needle, laser treatment, or treatment with light rays.
- Larger veins may be treated by injecting sclerosing agents into the vein. These substances in fact 'solidify' the vein so that it can no longer function.
- In more severe cases, there are various surgical treatments aimed at improving the blood flow in the veins; these procedures involve cutting out the problem major vein along its whole length.

12

Cellulite

Contents What is 'cellulite'? • Prevention of 'cellulite' • How NOT to treat 'cellulite' • Cosmetic preparations for 'cellulite' • Surgical methods for removing excess fat: liposuction

What is 'cellulite'?

The term 'cellulite' is widely used in everyday speech, but it has no scientific basis, and is not an accepted medical term.

Note: The reason the term 'cellulite' has a medical ring about it is that it sounds like the medical term 'cellulitis', but there is no connection between the two – **cellulitis** describes a bacterial infection of the skin.

So then, what does the term 'cellulite' mean? It refers to an unsightly distribution of fat under the skin, in certain areas of the body – especially the thighs and buttocks. The subcutaneous fat is distributed in a manner that creates hollows and bumps in these areas. This is in contrast to the uniform, smooth distribution of the subcutaneous fatty tissue in a young woman who is not overweight.

'Cellulite' is more common in women than in men, which suggests that it may be related to hormonal factors.

Why does 'cellulite' appear?

- The **sub-cutis**, which is composed mainly of fat , is found under the dermis.
- This layer of fat is made up of many fat cells that coalesce to form fatty tissue. These lumps of fat are surrounded and separated from each other by rigid strands.

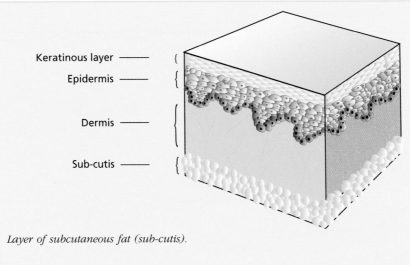

Keratinous layer

Epidermis

Dermis

Sub-cutis

Layer of subcutaneous fat (sub-cutis).

Subcutaneous fat divided into lumps by rigid strands.

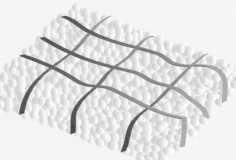

- If there is a high dietary intake of fats or carbohydrates (which are converted to fat in the body), the fat cells fill up with fat, swell up, and may grow to three or more times their normal size. On the other hand, the rigid strands cannot stretch beyond a certain amount. Thus the fatty tissue bulges out from the strands around it, which in turn tighten and restrict the fatty tissue even more, as shown in the illustration below.

Fatty tissue bulging out from the rigid strands that surround it.

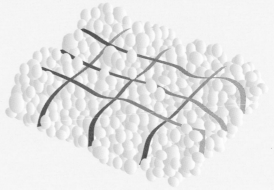

Prevention of 'cellulite'

Attention to diet/avoiding weight gain

Since good dietary habits prevent an increase in the amount of subcutaneous fat, there is a certain logic in this suggestion. Nevertheless, it must be remembered that 'cellulite' has a significant hereditary factor. There are some thin women who take great care with their diet but who still have cellulite.

It should be remembered that:

- a woman who has excess fat in the thighs and buttocks and goes on a reduction diet to lose weight may not necessarily lose fat from those particular areas;
- the loss of fat from areas that were bulging for a long period may result in **excess skin** that had previously been stretched over the fatty areas.

Therefore, it is important to adhere to sensible dietary habits over many years, to maintain a stable weight and to avoid weight gain. A 'crash' diet, to lose say 20 kilograms in 10 days, is undesirable – not only for the reasons mentioned above, but also for many other medical reasons.

Physical exercise

Physical exercise can further contribute and improve the appearance:

- by converting fat tissue to energy with subsequent decrease in excess fatty tissue;
- by increasing the bulk of the muscles – instead of the fat accumulating in large 'lumps', muscle tissue tends to grow in a uniform, smooth, more aesthetically acceptable manner.

How NOT to treat 'cellulite'

- It has not been shown scientifically that any dietary product can 'burn' and get rid of excess fat.
- Exercise machines that cause passive repeated movements of the fatty tissues of the thighs and buttocks so as to 'burn up' the fat have not proven to be effective.

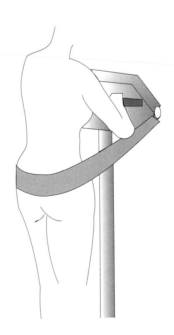

Exercise machine that causes passive movements of the fatty tissue.

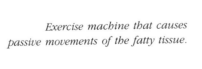

Cosmetic preparations for 'cellulite'

These products are supposed to penetrate through the keratin layer, the epidermis, and the dermis, and 'dissolve' the excess fatty tissue. The active ingredients commonly present in these preparations are methylxanthines or various plant extracts.

Methylxanthines

This group of substances are known to have a certain effect on fat cells. They break down and dissolve the fat in the cells. Substances in this group include:

- **theophylline**, which is derived from tea leaves, or produced synthetically;
- **caffeine**, which is present in coffee, tea, cola and guarana;
- **aminophylline**, which is used as a medication in asthma.

Note: It has not been proven scientifically or published in the accepted scientific literature that any product containing any of these substances can penetrate the subcutaneous tissues, 'dissolve' the fat and improve the texture of the tissues. From time to time, conflicting reports on the use of these substances are published.

Plant extracts

There is also no definite proof that any product that contains plant extracts has any effect. Some of these extracts contain substances similar in their chemical structure to the methylxanthines. Every now and then, a new product appears on the cosmetic scene, only to be supplanted by the next fad.

Surgical methods for removing excess fat: liposuction

In cases where the accumulation of subcutaneous fat is extreme, and causes psychological distress, one may consider referral for **liposuction**. In this procedure, a small incision (a few millimetres long) is made in the skin, a thin tube is inserted into the subcutaneous fat layer, and the fat cells are sucked out through the tube. Following liposuction, new fat cells will not grow or multiply in the area. If there is excessive plumpness in the area, it will be due to growth of those fat cells left behind, which accumulate more and more fat in them.

Not everybody is suitable to undergo liposuction, and an appropriately trained surgeon should be consulted with regard to the suitability for the operation, its advantages and disadvantages, and the expected outcome. It is difficult to predict the exact results following liposuction, and to a large extent the outcome depends on the skill of the surgeon.

Improvements in liposuction

There have been some new developments for improving the methods of lipo-suction. Among these is the transmission of sound waves into the tissue through a tube prior to sucking out the fat. This helps to dissolve and disinte-grate the fat tissue, making the suction process easier and more effective. It is worth mentioning that some doctors warn patients that the biological effects of activating sound waves on tissue at this intensity are not yet clear. The method is relatively new and its long-term effects (if there are any) may become known only years later.

13

Inflammation, dermatitis and cosmetics

Contents Overview • Definitions: inflammation and dermatitis • Stages in the development of skin inflammation • Causes and types of skin inflammation • Contact dermatitis • Types of contact dermatitis • Hypoallergenic preparations • Diagnosis • Principles of treatment

Overview

Cosmetics are a relatively common cause of skin inflammation: the inflammation results from exposure of the skin to a specific component (which may not always be identifiable) of the cosmetic preparation. To make this subject more easily understood, we first clarify what the term **inflammation** means; then we discuss the common types of skin inflammation. Finally, we discuss skin inflammations that result from contact with specific substances (including components of cosmetics).

Definitions: inflammation and dermatitis

The term **inflammation** can be defined simply as **the defensive response of the body to various processes, including infections (bacterial, viral or fungal), and many other injuries.** A chain of events, mainly involving the **white blood cells (leukocytes)**, results in the appearance of the inflammatory process. Inflammation is characterized by:

- **warmth** in the inflamed area;
- **redness** – due to dilatation of blood vessels;
- **swelling** – due to an increase in the permeability ('leakiness') of the blood vessels, with leakage of fluid;
- **pain** (or **itching**) – due to irritation of nerves;
- **loss of function** (partial or complete) of the involved organ or limb.

The term 'dermatitis' means inflammation of the skin. The term 'eczema' means the same as 'dermatitis' – they are synonymous.

Note: In general, in medical terminology, any inflammation is given the suffix -**itis**; for example inflammation of the appendix is called **appendicitis**, inflammation of the meninges (the coverings of the brain) is called **meningitis**, and inflammation of the dermis (skin) is called **dermatitis**.

Stages in the development of skin inflammation

Any inflammation of the skin, regardless of the cause, may appear at various stages. The accepted medical approach differentiates an **acute** phase from a **chronic** phase.

Acute phase
An acute illness, in medical terminology, is one that progresses rapidly, and does not last a long time (it either subsides or moves into a chronic phase). The skin in acute inflammation becomes red and swollen. In severe conditions, the skin may weep and blisters may appear.

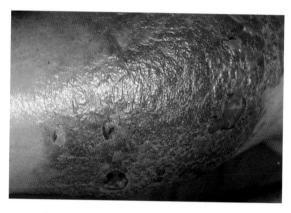

Acute skin inflammation.

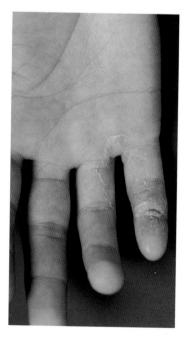

Chronic skin inflammation of a mechanic's hand following exposure to motor oils.

Chronic (prolonged) inflammation
This stage is characterized by a prolonged period of inflammation. The skin in chronic inflammation is dry, thickened and scaly, with accentuation of the normal skin markings; sometimes the skin is cracked.

Subacute inflammation

Another stage in the development of inflammation is the subacute phase. This is an intermediate stage, between acute and chronic. In subacute skin inflammation the skin is still red and swollen to a certain extent, but less so than in acute inflammation. There may be slight weeping. In certain areas the skin begins to peel.

Causes and types of skin inflammation

Skin inflammation can be due to a number of causes:

- infection
- diaper dermatitis
- seborrhoeic dermatitis
- atopic dermatitis
- contact dermatitis

We shall discuss **contact dermatitis** in more detail, since it may result from the use of cosmetic preparations.

Various types of skin inflammation

- **Skin infection**: any infection of the skin, bacterial, viral or fungal, produces a defensive response from the body, resulting in the appearance of inflammation.

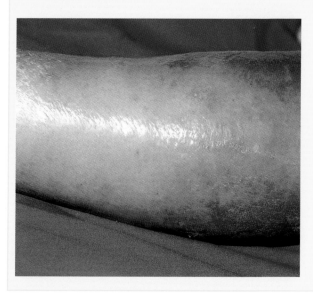

Infection in the leg: in the infected area, there are signs of inflammation, such as redness and swelling.

- **Diaper dermatitis**: this inflammation occurs in babies, in the diaper area, as a result of prolonged contact with urine and stool, or with remnants of soap or other substances that were applied to the area.
- **Seborrhoeic dermatitis**: this is an inflammatory process characterized by redness and scaling in specific areas; the areas that are usually affected by seborrhoeic dermatitis in adults are the scalp, the folds alongside the nose, and the eyebrows.
- **Atopic dermatitis**: this is a chronic skin inflammation that is related to hereditary factors, and manifested by dry skin, with marked itching. Atopic dermatitis is related to the group of allergic diseases called **atopic diseases**, which include asthma, allergic rhinitis ('hay fever') and allergic conjunctivitis (allergic eye inflammation).

We do not discuss the treatment of these conditions. In all such cases, the patient should seek medical attention.

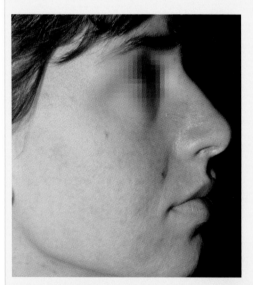

Seborrhoeic dermatitis.

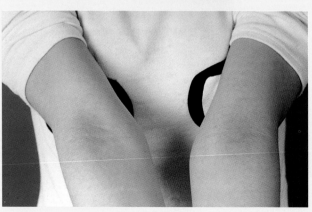

Atopic dermatitis.

Contact dermatitis

Overview

This common form of skin inflammation is caused by contact of certain substances with the skin. The skin is normally in contact with numerous substances, almost any of which can cause inflammation:

- by direct irritation of the skin – **irritant contact dermatitis**;
- by an allergic mechanism – **allergic contact dermatitis**.

Irritant contact dermatitis

In this case, the offending substance has a direct toxic effect on the skin. Hence the severity of the reaction depends on the concentration of the irritant substance and the period of exposure. This is not a specific sensitivity of a particular person to the substance: anybody coming in contact with that substance, above a certain concentration, and for a long enough time, will develop inflammation of the skin. For example, contact with various acids causes irritant contact dermatitis.

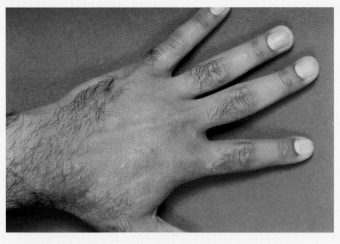

Irritant contact dermatitis following exposure to moderate concentrations of hydrochloric acid.

Allergic contact dermatitis

Allergy is a state of hypersensitivity arising from an immune response of the body to some substance. This can follow exposure to the substance by inhaling it, by swallowing it, or by direct contact of the substance with the skin. In allergic contact dermatitis, the allergic reaction occurs because of hypersensitivity to substances in direct contact with the skin.

Allergic contact dermatitis does not occur in everyone exposed to the specific substance

For some reason, partially due to a hereditary factor, there is a fault in the patient's immune response. In an allergic patient, the immune system is triggered by a substance that normally has no adverse effects, but in that specific patient causes an inflammatory response of the skin. In the classic and most common form of allergic contact dermatitis, the patient has been exposed to the same offending substance for long periods in the past without developing any reaction. During this period, however, an unnoticed process occurs and an allergic response develops in the body's immune system. At a certain stage, the response becomes manifest, and, from then on, every exposure to the substance may be followed by an allergic response.

The offending substance may be a cleansing agent, any cosmetic preparation, a metal such as nickel or chrome, glues, etc. Once the immune system has been able to identify and react against a certain substance, the allergic reaction can occur following exposure to minute amounts of the substance; the patient does not need to come into contact with a large amount of the substance to develop an allergic reaction. Furthermore, there does not have to be daily exposure to the substance to produce an allergic reaction: infrequent exposure – even once every few weeks or years – to small amounts of the substance may be sufficient to trigger such a reaction.

Types of contact dermatitis

Hand eczema

This is a common problem, and is the result of prolonged exposure to water and cleaning agents, to which housewives and other workers (e.g. food handlers, florists) are frequently subject. Prolonged exposure to cleaning agents removes the oily layer of the skin surface. The combination of this loss of the oily protective layer with frequent exposure to cleaning agents that may contain irritant and/or allergenic substances results in hand **eczema** (or 'hand dermatitis'), sometimes called '**housewife's eczema**'. The chronic form of hand eczema is manifested by the appearance of scaling and fissures.

From time to time, there may be flare-ups of acute inflammation, with reddening and swelling of the skin.

This inflammation occurs on the palms, backs of the hands, webs of the fingers, and underneath rings, bracelets and watch straps, because remnants of cleaning agents and other offending materials tend to remain there, with subsequent prolonged contact with the skin.

Usually some improvement can be observed if the patient refrains from cleaning activities. The inflammation recurs on resuming these activities without appropriate protection.

Potassium dichromate, nickel and other allergens

Detergents frequently contain a substance called potassium dichromate, which penetrates the skin and causes contact dermatitis. Potassium dichromate gets into the cleaning agents during their manufacture, although it plays no role in the cleaning actions. There are cleaning agents that do not contain potassium dichromate. In many other cases, the sensitivity is triggered by nickel – a metal that is a very common component in rings, bracelets and watch straps. Wetting the skin results in the release of very small quantities of nickel, which comes into contact with the skin and causes allergic contact dermatitis.

In addition, certain common foodstuffs, especially vegetables and fruits, may provoke allergic reactions.

Prevention of hand eczema

Contact with water and detergents should be avoided as much as possible. As explained in Chapter 4 on skin moisture and moisturizers, repeated exposure to water dries the skin. In addition, detergents are designed to remove the layer of grease from the dishes, but by the same token they remove the protective oily skin layer that coats the skin and protects it. To minimize contact with water and detergents, it is advisable to adopt the following measures.

- Gloves should be worn.

Note: The rubber of normal gloves may itself contain substances that can trigger an allergic skin reaction. Furthermore, so long as one wears rubber gloves, the hands are constantly moist as a result of small amounts of water that may have got into the glove and from perspiration. It is important to use gloves that have an inner lining made of cotton, or to wear an inner set of cotton gloves underneath the rubber ones. In any case, the rubber gloves should be worn for as brief a period as possible (and for no longer than a few minutes). If it is felt that the hands are perspiring, the gloves should be removed and the hands 'aired'.

- Advantage should be taken of appliances such as dishwashers and washing machines (or other members of the family!).

- Occlusive ointments should be applied frequently in order to isolate the skin from cleansing agents. Silicone-containing preparations may be used as well. Details of silicone preparations appear in Chapter 4 on skin moisture and moisturizers. However, if there is skin inflammation, protective preparations should not be applied. In this case, the first thing to do is to seek medical advice for treatment of the inflammation. Only after the inflammation has disappeared should protective cream be applied.

- In cases where an association between hand dermatitis and certain foodstuffs is identified, contact with these substances should be avoided as much as possible.

Hand eczema can be a form of atopic dermatitis

Note that, infrequently, hand eczema is not related to contact with offending substances. Sometimes, it represents a unique form of **atopic dermatitis**. These cases are much more difficult to deal with, and the commonly accepted modalities of prevention and treatment are not so effective.

Treatment of hand eczema
See Chapter 20 on preparations used in dermatology.

Phytodermatitis and phytophotodermatitis

Contact dermatitis can be caused by contact with plants, flowers, or fruit juices. This phenomenon is called **phytodermatitis** (Greek: *phyton* = plant).

In other cases, the actual contact with the plant does not cause skin inflammation. The allergic reaction occurs only after the skin has been exposed to sunlight. This phenomenon is known as **phytophotodermatitis**.

Plants known to cause these reactions include chrysanthemums, celery, mango, citrus fruits, figs and others.

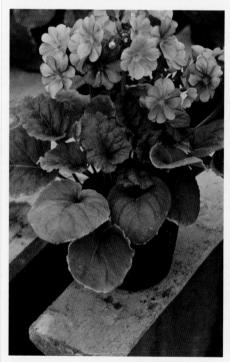

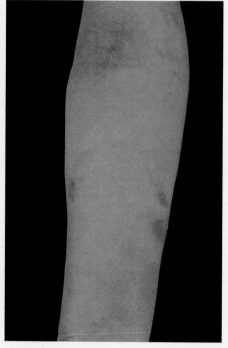

Primula obconica: *skin inflammation may appear after touching the dry petals of the plant.*

Skin inflammation following exposure to Primula obconica.

Cosmetics and dermatitis

Cosmetics can cause contact dermatitis. The chances of this happening are relatively low, considering the number of people using cosmetics, but it does occur. It is estimated that about 10% of women who use cosmetics develop contact dermatitis from some cosmetic preparation at least once in their lives.

Cosmetic preparations contain several components, any one of which could potentially cause skin inflammation:

- the active ingredient of the preparation
- the vehicle (base) that contains the active ingredient
- additional components that may be present, such as fragrances or preservatives

Before using any cosmetic preparation it is important to establish that the user is not allergic to one of its components. Before using some cosmetic for the first time, some should be applied to a small area of skin that is not exposed (usually behind the ear) for a few days. Only after confirming that there is no intolerance should the preparation be used regularly. It should be remembered, however, that sensitivity can appear with time – even to a substance that has been used frequently.

If sensitivity to a specific preparation appears:
1 Use of the preparation should be discontinued.
2 A dermatologist's advice should be sought, and he/she should be consulted as to how the particular component of the preparation that was responsible can be identified. Subsequently, preparations containing that specific chemical should be avoided.

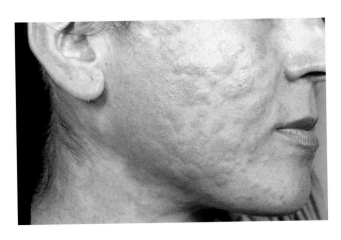

Allergic contact dermatitis following exposure to fragrance in a facial moisturizer.

Hypoallergenic preparations

Hypoallergenic preparations usually do not contain components such as perfumes or certain preservatives that statistically are known to have a higher than average risk of causing allergic reactions.

Note: It should not be forgotten that hypoallergenic preparations can still cause allergy.

Sensitivity to a particular substance is an individual characteristic. In practice, there is no cosmetic preparation that can never cause an allergic reaction in someone.

The term 'hypoallergenic' may be misleading. Many people mistakenly believe that such preparations do not contain any substance that can cause an allergic reaction. However, hypoallergenic preparations can also contain various fragrances, preservatives and other components that may also induce an allergic reaction. Nevertheless, statistically, the likelihood of a hypoallergenic preparation causing an allergic reaction is certainly less than that of a normal preparation.

Diagnosis

Usually, the most efficient way of diagnosing the cause of the inflammation is by questioning the patient carefully. In some cases, the patient has a fairly good idea what caused the problem, and will tell you that the rash appeared after using a certain cosmetic or medical preparation. However, the offending agent may be present in many different cosmetic preparations. Therefore avoiding the use of one particular preparation and replacing it with another may not necessarily solve the problem.

To identify precisely to which particular component the patient has reacted, there is a special test kit called a **'patch test'**. In this test, substances known to commonly cause allergic reactions are applied to an area of clean, unaffected skin

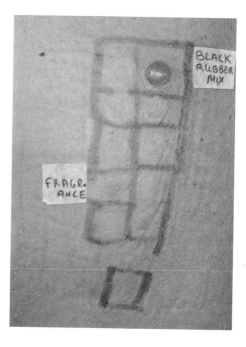

Patch test demonstrating sensitivity to black rubber. In this case, the patient should avoid contact with rubber products.

(usually the skin of the back). The substances are applied on small discs that are held against the patient's skin with special adhesive plaster. From 48 to 96 hours later, if the patient is indeed allergic to one or more of the test substances, a skin inflammation will appear at the area of contact (under that specific disc). The inflammation is manifested by redness, itching and sometimes the appearance of blisters, depending on the level of sensitivity to the material being tested.

Skin allergy to cosmetics can be a prolonged, frustrating problem. The treatment requires patience. Having diagnosed the offending substance by the patch test, one then has to embark on a process (often lengthy and tedious) of finding cosmetic preparations that do not contain that substance or other substances that are chemically similar to it.

Principles of treatment

Prevention

Treatment is based first and foremost on prevention. If it is known what the substance is that caused the reaction then contact of that substance with the skin should be avoided.

Corticosteroids

The most effective treatment for dermatitis involves the use of corticosteroid preparations for application to the skin. Steroids are very effective at suppressing inflammation. The dermatologist has at his/her disposal a wide range of such preparations, of varying strengths for differing degrees of inflammation. These preparations should be given on a physician's advice, and must never be used for self-medication; most are only available on a doctor's prescription. Only preparations that contain low concentrations of hydrocortisone (0.5–1%) may be purchased over the counter in the USA. The use of corticosteroids is discussed in detail in Chapter 20 on preparations used in dermatology.

In more severe cases of inflammation, oral medications (e.g. tablets) containing corticosteroids are sometimes necessary, and may even be given by intramuscular injection.

Antihistamines

Allergic skin reactions involve the release of **histamine** in the affected tissues, with subsequent exacerbation of the inflammatory reaction; therefore **antihistamine medications** may be used to lessen the allergic response. Antihistamine preparations may be applied to the skin as creams or gels. However, these preparations themselves may cause allergic reactions; hence some physicians recommend patients to avoid the use of topical antihistamines.

Oral antihistamine preparations are used in various inflammatory situations (including allergic processes that occur in the skin). Some of these medications require a doctor's prescription.

Note: Some antihistamine medications may cause drowsiness and fatigue. Therefore there are strict restrictions regarding driving a motor vehicle after taking them. This also applies to engaging in any other activity in which decreased alertness may be dangerous. A physician should be consulted before an antihistamine is taken.

Other treatments

Other types of treatment are available, such as phototherapy (in which the skin is exposed to ultraviolet rays) and may be used at the physician's discretion.

14

Skin tumours

Contents Overview • Basic definitions • What types of tumours occur
in the skin? • Skin tumours that originate in the keratinocytes • Skin
tumours that originate in the melanocytes • Prevention • Self-examination
• Regular medical examinations • Management of possibly cancerous
lesions

Overview

It is very important for a cosmetician to have a basic knowledge of skin
tumours. Clients may ask cosmeticians many questions relating to skin
tumours; in the course of their professional work, cosmeticians may come
across a variety of skin lesions and growths. In this chapter, we define some
basic terms related to tumours in general, and present the main features of
some of the more common skin tumours.

Note: This chapter is not intended to grant cosmeticians qualification to treat
skin tumours. However, a better knowledge and understanding of this topic
can provide the reader with the tools to recognize common skin tumours,
and in particular, to identify abnormal lesions that require referral of the
client to a dermatologist.

A skin lesion is actually any abnormal condition that appears on the skin.
Dermatology is the science of diagnosing and treating skin lesions. There are
many reasons for lesions to appear on the skin: they may be infectious (due to
viruses, bacteria or fungi); there are inflammatory lesions; and there are
tumourous lesions – growths of the skin – which is what this chapter will deal
with.

Basic definitions

Below are some of the basic definitions in the field of skin tumours. A **tumour**
(= **growth** = **neoplasm**) is a lesion that represents an abnormal overgrowth of
body tissue. This overgrowth results from uncontrolled proliferation of the
tumour cells.

The formation of a tumour

The tumorous process results from a change in the genetic features of a certain cell. A change in the genetic content of a cell can lead to repeated divisions and replications of that cell, with its abnormal proliferation, as shown in the diagram.

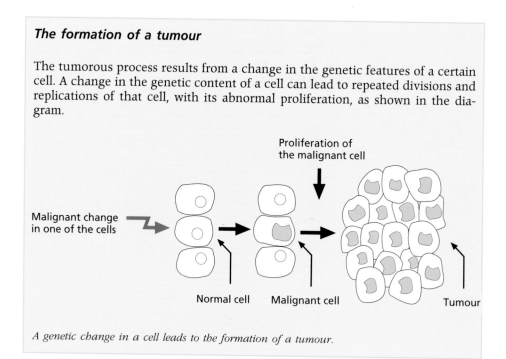

A genetic change in a cell leads to the formation of a tumour.

A tumour may be benign or malignant. A **benign tumour** does not spread aggressively. It remains limited to the region in which it formed; it has defined borders that can be clearly distinguished from their surroundings.

Note: It should be clarified that while the word 'tumour' or 'growth' in everyday use has a frightening connotation, in medical/scientific terminology, a wide range of lesions are classified as benign tumours. For example, in medical/scientific terminology, a melanocytic naevus ('mole', 'beauty mark') is defined as a benign tumour. In spite of that frightening-sounding name, obviously, moles are considered common skin lesions that have no particular medical implications. Nevertheless, the presence of moles requires regular medical follow-up, in order to ascertain that they remain normal and do not develop any suspicious changes.

In contrast, a **malignant tumour** tends to spread aggressively. The tumour cells divide and replicate uncontrollably, and the body's defence mechanisms are unable to halt or control the cell division. The edges of a malignant tumour are not well defined, and cannot be clearly identified, since the tumour cells invade and destroy the surrounding tissues.

Tumour cells that spread to distant areas of the body, remote from the primary tumour, are called metastases.

What are metastases?

A **metastasis** (plural: **metastases**) is a group of malignant cells that have broken away from the primary, original tumour and have found their way to other tissues

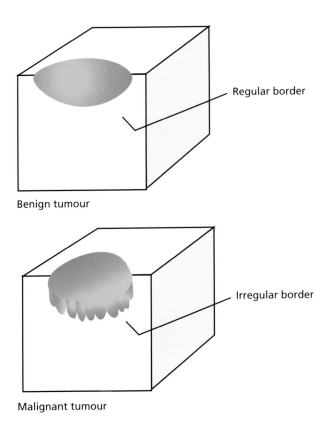

Regular border

Benign tumour

Irregular border

Malignant tumour

Benign versus malignant tumour: diagrammatic representation.

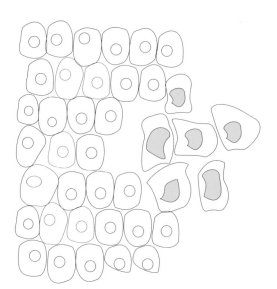

Local spread of a malignant tumour: direct extension of the malignant cells (marked in yellow) into the surrounding tissues.

in the body. In those tissues, which may be close to the original (primary) tumour or far from it, the malignant cells continue to divide and cause destruction. The tumour cells can spread, for example, by way of the lymphatic system or the bloodstream. In this way, malignant cells originating in a tumour can reach various organs in the body via the bloodstream. They can reach, for example, the liver, brain, lungs, bones and other organs. The cause of death from malignancies is frequently related to the presence of metastases in various internal organs, and the damage to those organs wreaked by the metastases. The development of metastases is therefore the hallmark of malignant tumours; **there are no metastases from benign tumours**.

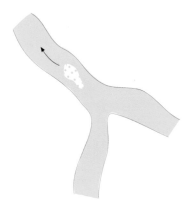

Tumour cells are carried in the blood vessels to distant sites (metastases).

The progress of a malignant tumour in summary
- A genetic change takes place in a single cell.
- Repeated cell divisions of that particular cell will result in a malignant tumour that continues growing, until it may eventually become visible to the naked eye.
- Cells from the tumour can break away from the original mass, and establish themselves (as metastases) in distant tissues, with subsequent destruction of those tissues.

The term 'cancer' means exactly the same as 'malignant tumour'
The word 'cancer', which is Latin for 'crab', is apparently related to the resemblance of the malignant cells spreading out of the primary tumour in the shape of a crab. While the term 'cancer' is widely used in everyday language, 'malignant tumour' is the accepted medical/scientific term.

What is the source of tumours in the human body?
Every cell in the body, including skin cells, can potentially develop into a tumour. In any cell, a possible 'fault' may occur, which will trigger an abnormal division of that particular cell. This abnormal cell division may be limited, in which case a benign tumour results, or it may be uncontrolled, overwhelming the body's defence systems, and resulting in a malignant tumour.

What types of tumours occur in the skin?

A skin tumour may develop from any of the living cells present in the skin, i.e. the source of the tumour may be in the epidermis, dermis or the sub-cutis.

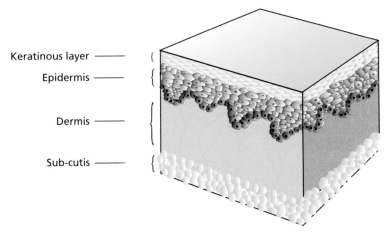

Keratinous layer ——

Epidermis ——

Dermis ——

Sub-cutis ——

Diagram of the structure of the skin.

Epidermis
Most of the skin tumours to be described in this chapter arise from the epidermis. The main cell in the epidermis is the **keratinocyte**, or **squamous cell**, which may be the origin of a tumour. In addition, there are other cells in the epidermis, for example **melanocytes**. These latter cells produce the pigment melanin (you will recall that melanin is the major determinant of skin colour). Melanocytes can be the source of various growths as well.

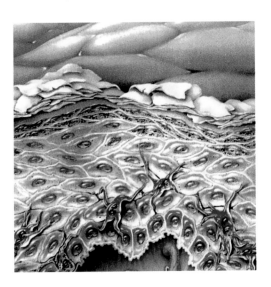

Melanocytes (red) in the basal layer of the epidermis.

Dermis

The dermis contains:

- sebaceous glands
- sweat glands
- nerve cells
- blood vessels
- muscle cells
- other types of cells and tissues

Any of these may be the source of a skin tumour. Such tumours may be benign or malignant. In addition, metastases from primary malignant tumours in other parts of the body may get to the skin. For example, a malignant tumour of the lung or the breast may seed metastases that will get to the skin and present as lumps in the skin.

In this chapter, we discuss only the relatively common skin tumours.

There are two important messages that arise from this chapter, with regard to the diagnosis of skin tumours:

- Any injury or lesion of the skin that persists for a long time (weeks or months) must be suspected as a possible cancer. Common examples of this kind of problem are squamous cell carcinoma and basal cell carcinoma – discussed in two of the boxes later in this chapter.
- It is important to know how to recognize a 'normal' mole and an 'abnormal' mole – details are given later in this chapter.

Skin tumours that originate in the keratinocytes

These are:

- solar keratosis (a precancerous lesion)
- squamous cell carcinoma
- basal cell carcinoma

Note: Both basal cell carcinoma and squamous cell carcinoma are defined as 'cancerous' growths. The term **carcinoma** covers a wide range of malignant tumours of various types.

Solar keratosis

In general, the term **keratosis** means a thickening of the keratinous layer of the skin. This thickening is seen in various inflammatory processes that occur in the skin, but can also be a cancerous or precancerous condition, as in solar keratosis. These lesions usually occur in fair-skinned people over the age of 40. They appear in areas exposed to the sun – the face and the backs of the hands. They are slightly raised, dry, rough, pink–red lesions, with a slightly scaly surface. These lesions originate from the keratinocytes in the epidermis. Keratinocytes are also called **squamous cells**.

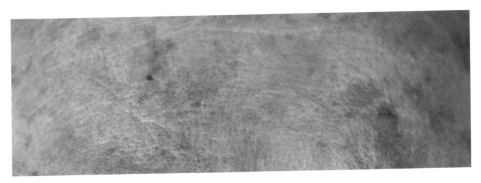

Solar keratoses on sun-damaged skin.

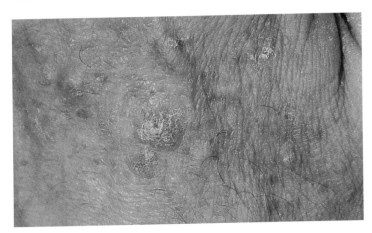

Several small keratoses on the back of the hand of an elderly man.

A solar keratosis is a **precancerous lesion**; that is to say, it is still not considered malignant. Having said that, if the lesion extends beyond the epidermis and reaches the dermis (as shown in the figure on the right), it in fact becomes a **squamous cell carcinoma**, and is then defined as a cancerous skin lesion.

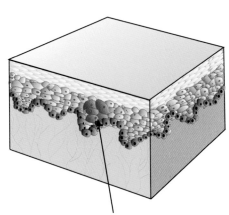

Development of solar keratoses from epidermal keratinocytes.

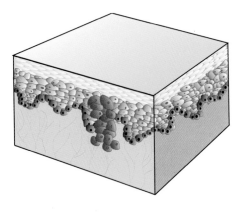

*Some cells of the solar keratosis have broken through into the dermis. The lesion is now considered a **squamous cell carcinoma**.*

Treatment of solar keratosis

Although the likelihood of a solar keratosis turning into a cancer is statistically extremely low, the lesion must be treated by a physician. The treatment is based on destroying the lesion – there is usually no need to excise it surgically. There are a number of methods available to the doctor. The most widely used are:

- freezing the lesion with liquid nitrogen, which destroys the cells of the lesion;
- treatment with a preparation for local use, called 5-FU (5-fluorouracil), which is available as a cream. This substance has the ability to reach and concentrate specifically in the abnormal cells, and destroy them.

Note: Sometimes the lesion cannot be definitely identified, and the doctor may not be fully convinced that it is indeed a solar keratosis. If there is any doubt, and the lesion may be some other skin tumour, it should be excised in its entirety and examined under the microscope.

Squamous cell carcinoma

As in solar keratosis, squamous cell carcinoma arises from keratinocytes (squamous cells) in the epidermis, except that in this case the tumour does not remain confined to the epidermis, but spreads into the dermis (as shown in the illustration earlier). Sometimes the tumour spreads even further, into deeper tissues, and may even seed metastases to internal body organs.

Squamous cell carcinoma may appear on normal-looking skin, or it may arise from solar keratoses.

This tumour usually appears in later life. In most cases, it arises in areas of skin exposed to the sun, but it can appear in areas that are not normally exposed. Indeed, squamous cell carcinoma can arise inside the mouth.

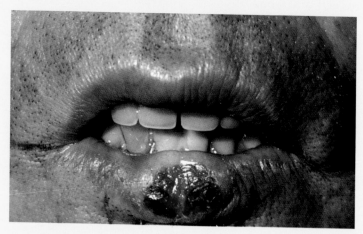

Squamous cell carcinoma of the lower lip: this is a very common site for squamous cell carcinoma to appear.

The tumour usually looks like a 'sore' on the skin; in other words, in the area of the tumour the normal skin is absent, exposing the underlying tissues to varying degrees. Since the tumour tissue has destroyed the normal protective skin layers, the area of the tumour may become infected with bacteria, and a purulent (pus) discharge may appear. The characteristic feature that helps to distinguish this tumour from an innocent sore is the time factor. Any sore that does not heal within a reasonable time – a few weeks – requires urgent referral to a dermatologist.

This tumour can also appear as a lump above the skin level, commonly slightly 'damaged' on its surface. Other forms of squamous cell carcinoma may occur as well.

Basal cell carcinoma = basalioma = BCC

In this case, the renegade cells that have multiplied and produced a tumour originate from the keratinocytes in the basal layer of the epidermis.

Basal cell carcinoma is a common skin tumour. As with solar keratosis and squamous cell carcinoma, the direct cause of this tumour is prolonged, cumulative exposure to the sun. The lesions usually appear in people of light complexion, over the age of 40, and in areas exposed to the sun, including the nose, ears, bald areas of the scalp, neck, upper chest, and back. Basal cell carcinoma has a low degree of malignancy. It is very rare for a BCC to seed metastases. Although it grows slowly, in its original location it may cause marked destruction of the surrounding tissues. After a long time, the tumour may penetrate the soft tissues under the skin, and may even penetrate underlying bones. Hence, if a BCC is not treated early and completely excised, at a later stage a much larger tumour will need to be treated by losing a much larger area of the affected skin.

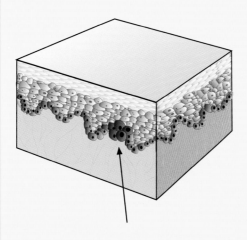

The basal layer of the epidermis, where basal cell carcinoma starts to develop.

Continued

A basal cell carcinoma is most commonly manifested as follows: a small, shiny swelling appears in an area exposed to the sun. The lesion slowly grows larger. Usually there are tiny blood vessels visible over its surface. A typical lesion usually develops elevated margins, whose colour is commonly referred to in medical texts as 'pearly'. Later, the tumour tissue destroys the normal skin tissues in the area, and a 'sore' appears in the centre.

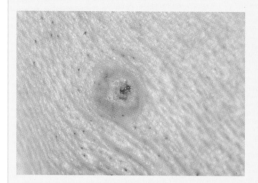
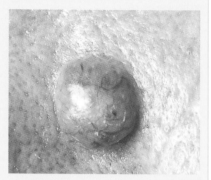

Basal cell carcinoma: the 'pearly' margins surround a typical sore.

Basal cell carcinoma; blood vessels are seen over its surface.

Although the above is the commonest presentation of a basal cell carcinoma, other forms may occur.

Note: Whenever a skin 'injury' or sore does not heal for a relatively long time (several weeks), the possibility of basal cell carcinoma or squamous cell carcinoma should be considered, and the client should be referred to a doctor as soon as possible.

Skin tumours that originate in the melanocytes

These include:

- melanocytic naevi ('moles', 'beauty marks')
- malignant melanoma

A naevus is a common skin lesion that is considered benign. As long as the naevus remains 'normal', there is no medical problem (this will be discussed in more detail below). On the other hand, **a melanoma is a very aggressive malignant tumour**. If not identified and treated early, melanoma tends to metastasize throughout the body, and it is considered a highly dangerous and potentially disastrous lesion. In recent years, the incidence of malignant melanoma has been increasing.

Note: Skin tumours originating from melanocytes are usually dark in colour – brown, bluish, or black. However, a few cases are not pigmented. On the other hand, tumours arising from keratinocytes are usually light-coloured, and rarely dark.

There are other skin lesions derived from melanocytes: solar lentigines ('sun spots') and freckles are discussed in more detail in Chapter 18 on bleaching.

Melanocytic naevus ('mole')

This lesion originates from the melanocyte, the cell that produces the pigment melanin in the epidermis.

In this case, the growth and proliferation of the melanocytes is **controlled**. The lesion is benign – scientifically, a mole is by definition a benign tumour. Because it is such a common lesion, the connotations of the term 'tumour' do not really apply to a mole.

In general, moles develop gradually, usually within the first 20 years of life; only 3–4% of newborn infants have moles. The number of moles gradually increases until about the age of 25, so that most people have some moles somewhere on their skin.

There are several different types of moles. They may be raised or flat, and their colour may vary from light brown to dark brown. If a lesion is indeed benign, it is expected to have a regular, clearly defined edge and uniform colour over its entire surface. It is important to be sure that a lesion is, in fact, a benign mole, and one must distinguish an innocent, normal mole from one where atypical changes are taking place or one that shows unusual features. Changes in the appearance of a mole could suggest the diagnosis of malignant melanoma, which necessitates the removal of the mole so that it can be examined under the microscope.

Changes in a mole that are suggestive of malignancy, and should turn on a 'warning light'

These include:

- irregular, poorly defined edges
- non-uniform colouration
- asymmetry
- rapid growth
- bleeding or discharge from a mole; the appearance of a 'sore' within a mole

These changes do not necessarily mean that the mole (naevus) is malignant. There are perfectly innocent moles whose coloration is not uniform, and similarly a lesion may bleed for any one of a number of simple, banal reasons. Nevertheless, if there is any doubt, the patient must be referred urgently to an experienced physician.

The above changes are dealt with in more detail in the section below on malignant melanoma.

Malignant melanoma

This is the most aggressive skin cancer, with the highest mortality rate. There has been a gradual increase in its incidence. The likelihood of a light-skinned person developing malignant melanoma in his/her lifetime is estimated today at almost 1%. There is substantial evidence that someone who was exposed intensively to sunlight in the past, such as to have caused a sunburn, is at much higher risk of developing melanoma. We are not talking here just of prolonged, cumulative exposure. A severe sunburn in childhood or adolescence significantly increases one's risk of developing melanoma later in life.

The source of melanoma is the cell that produces melanin in the epidermis – the **melanocyte**. Hence a melanoma is usually (but not necessarily) brown/black/blue in colour.

If the tumour is diagnosed at an early stage and is completely removed, with a safety margin of surrounding healthy skin, complete recovery can be expected. On the other hand, if the tumour is not diagnosed in time, and has penetrated deeper into the skin, it will almost certainly have metastasized to other areas of the patient's body, and the outcome will be fatal.

Medicine has yet to find a cure for melanoma that has penetrated a certain distance into the dermis. Such a melanoma will almost certainly seed malignant metastases to distant tissues of the body and eventually result in death.

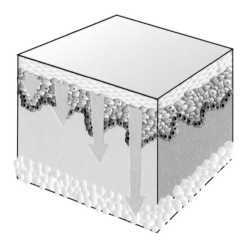

The deeper the melanoma penetrates into the dermis, the worse is the outcome.

A malignant melanoma can develop from a melanocytic naevus ('mole') or from skin that has been damaged by cumulative exposure to the sun, or it may appear 'de novo', from healthy skin.

When should you suspect that a lesion is not just an ordinary 'innocent' mole, but one that may be a melanoma?

Irregular, poorly defined edges

This is when the edges of the lesion partly blend into the surrounding skin, and you cannot see a definite border between the mole and the healthy skin. In addition, any change in the appearance of the border – such as from a round border to a jagged one – should arouse your suspicion.

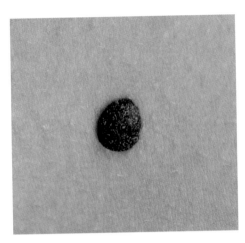 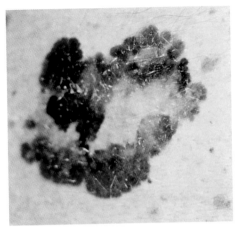

Note the poorly defined border of the lesion shown on the right, which was diagnosed as melanoma. Compare that with the clearly seen sharp border between the skin and the lesion shown on the left, which is of a benign mole.

Non-uniform coloration

A non-uniform colour of the lesion, or the development of other colours within the lesion – blue, grey, red or, in particular, a deep, black hue – indicate a lesion that is developing abnormally. Also, the appearance of islands of 'normal' skin within a dark lesion should arouse suspicion.

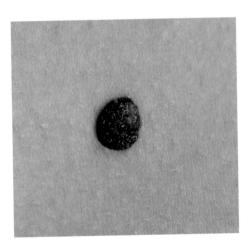 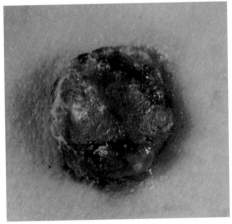

Note the non-uniform colour of the lesion shown on the right, which was diagnosed as melanoma. Compare that with the uniform colouration of the lesion shown on the left, which is a benign mole.

Asymmetry of the lesion

This is a suspicious sign; in contrast to the symmetric, regular shapes of innocent moles.

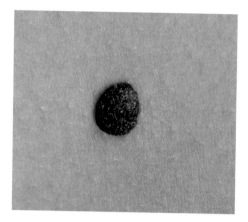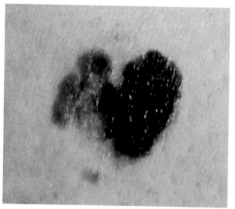

Note the asymmetric shape of the melanoma shown on the right, in contrast to the symmetric shape of the benign mole shown on the left.

Unusually rapid growth

In children and adolescents, moles generally grow in parallel to the overall growth of the child. A lesion that seems to be growing out of proportion to the child's general growth should arouse suspicion. Therefore a sudden acceleration in the growth rate of a lesion is worrisome. In an adult, any skin lesion that seems to be growing should be seen by a doctor.

Bleeding or discharge from a mole or the appearance of a sore within it

Any abnormal, uncharacteristic course of a naevus (including the onset of itching or pain) should arouse suspicion, and the patient should be examined by a doctor.

Note: The appearance of a relatively large lesion (above 6 mm diameter) is also considered to be a suspicious sign. However, that does not mean that 'small' lesions may be ignored. There have been melanomas as small as 2 or 3 mm. **In any case of a suspicious lesion, refer the client urgently to an experienced physician!**

Prevention

Early detection is of paramount importance. The simplest way to diagnose a malignant lesion early is by self-examination.

Self-examination

Self-examination is carried out in front of a mirror. It must include all areas of the body, including 'hidden' areas that one tends to overlook, such as the buttocks, soles of the feet and the genital region.

How to carry out a self-examination

In front of a mirror
This part of the examination covers the face (including inside the mouth), the neck and chest; women should lift up their breasts to examine the skin underneath. The armpits should be examined. The mirror is used to examine all the areas of the upper arms, forearms, thighs and lower legs.

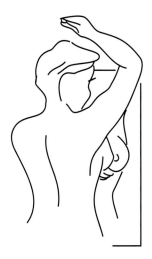

Self-examination in front of a mirror.

Using a second mirror
The ears, behind the ears, the back of the neck, shoulders and upper back should be examined. The second mirror should also be used to examine the lower back, the buttocks and the back of the legs.

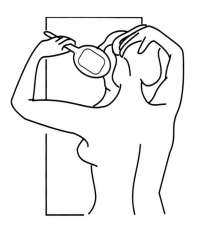

Using a second mirror.

The scalp
The scalp can be examined with the assistance of a second person – a friend or member of the family. A hairdryer is useful to spread the hair out and expose all areas of the scalp.

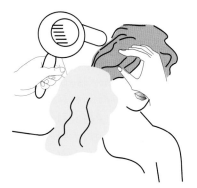

Examining the scalp using a hairdryer.

The following areas should be carefully examined:
- hands – palms and backs of the hands, between the fingers, and under the fingernails
- genitalia
- the legs and soles (it is easiest to do this while sitting, using a stool)

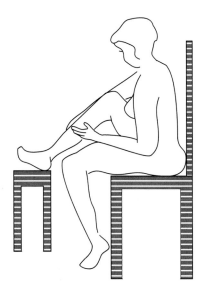

Examining the soles.

Regular medical examinations

A regular check-up by a doctor should be scheduled every few months. The more risk factors a person has for skin malignancies, the more frequent these examinations should be. The major risk factors requiring more frequent check-ups are:

- fair complexion
- a past history of a melanoma or skin cancer
- a family history of melanoma or skin cancer

Management of possibly cancerous lesions

If any of the lesions described above – squamous cell carcinoma, basal cell carcinoma, a suspicious mole or malignant melanoma – is found, the physician must remove it in its entirety, with a 'safety margin' of surrounding normal-looking skin.

Note: A lesion suspected of being cancerous should not be treated by methods that will destroy it and not enable it to be examined under the microscope (such as 'freezing' the lesion with liquid nitrogen, burning it off (cauterization) with an electric needle, or destroying it by using local chemical preparations). A skin lesion may only be treated with one of those techniques if an experienced doctor has diagnosed it and determined that cauterization is the appropriate treatment (for example, solar keratoses may be treated by liquid nitrogen).

Every lesion that is suspected of being cancerous must be examined microscopically. The removal of any piece of tissue from the body, including skin, for the purpose of laboratory examination is called a **biopsy**. There are several reasons for performing a biopsy:

1 To make a definitive diagnosis regarding the type of a tumour (since this diagnosis will determine the proper treatment);
2 To confirm that the tumour has been completely removed, and that no tumour tissue (or malignant cells) remains in, or under, the patient's skin;
3 To determine the depth to which the tumour has reached: in many cases, the depth of the tumour has prognostic implications, i.e. it allows prediction of the probable future course of the illness; the depth is also a factor that determines the proper treatment.

Note: The pharmaceutical industry produces chemical substances that cause localized destruction of skin tissue. These substances can be purchased only with a doctor's prescription, and only a doctor may use them. If a tumour has been cauterized (burnt off) or treated by local application of a chemical substance, or not removed in its entirety, the area of the lesion may heal, and may be covered by scar tissue – **but underneath the scar there will still be tumour cells**. These residual tumour cells may proliferate and give rise later to a cancerous state, with severe consequences for the patient. Therefore **only an experienced physician can determine the type of treatment that is appropriate for skin lesions**. In any case, 'amateur' treatment of skin lesions with chemicals should be avoided. Such treatment may only be carried out by an experienced physician.

How does a surgeon remove a suspected cancerous lesion from the skin?
In the case of a skin lesion that is suspected of being malignant (such as a basal cell carcinoma, squamous cell carcinoma, or malignant melanoma), an **excisional biopsy** is performed – that is, the surgeon biopsies the lesion after removing it in its entirety.

Steps in the procedure

1 **Anaesthesia**: Local anaesthetic is injected into the area of the lesion.

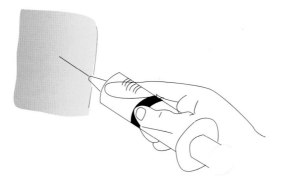

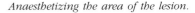
Anaesthetizing the area of the lesion.

2 **Excising the lesion**: The physician uses a **scalpel** – a surgical knife. The commonly used incision is lens-shaped, which is usually the most effective and easiest shape for total removal of a lesion. The incision should also include a rim of healthy tissue around the lesion, so as to ensure total removal of all the cells of the lesion. Sometimes, because of the shape or location of the lesion a lens-shaped incision cannot be used, and some other shape of incision should be carried out.

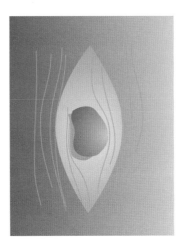

'Lens-shaped' incision around a lesion.

3 **Suturing the surgical wound**: Suture is used for sewing up the incision. The stitches are removed some days later, the exact time depending mainly on the size and location of the incision. In places where the skin is delicate and cannot be put under tension, such as the skin of the face, the stitches are removed after five to seven days. In places where the skin is thick (areas where the skin is normally subjected to various forces in the course of normal activities), such as the back or the limbs, the stitches are removed after ten to fourteen days.

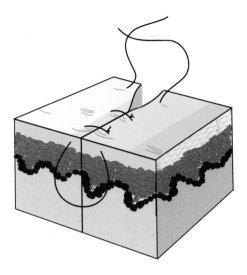

Suturing the surgical incision.

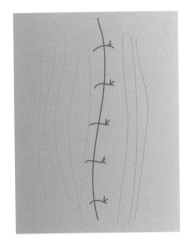

After suturing the surgical incision.

4 **The excised skin is sent for microscopic diagnosis of the lesion**: Once the type of lesion and its depth have been determined, it is possible to determine if the excisional biopsy that was carried out will suffice, or whether further treatment may be necessary.

In the case of a malignant melanoma, other treatments may be necessary:

- Further excision of the skin surrounding the excised lesion – creating wider 'safety' margins – may be performed.
- Removal of adjacent lymph nodes may be considered.
- In severe cases, chemotherapy may be considered, i.e. anti-cancer drugs may be given in an attempt to destroy tumour cells in distant areas.

Summary
The treatment of skin lesions suspected of being cancerous is based on total removal of the lesion, with 'safety margins' of normal skin surrounding the lesion. Such lesions must never be burnt off with an electric cautery needle, or destroyed by the application of chemical substances. Every case of a suspected cancerous skin lesion must be referred to an experienced physician.

15

Active ingredients in cosmetic preparations

Contents Overview • Naturally occurring substances extracted from animal tissues • Plant extracts • Vitamins • Common foodstuffs • Some additional comments

Overview

Recently there have been significant developments in the cosmetics industry. The general trend of the industry is towards improving the health of the skin, and not merely improving its appearance temporarily. Many preparations for skin care lie in the grey area between cosmetics and drugs. This chapter reviews the various active ingredients in cosmetic preparations, and what we know regarding their actions and effects. The following discussion is based on accredited scientific research and the results published in the scientific and medical literature. Research is also carried out by the leading cosmetics companies; however, the results are published infrequently and the information is not readily accessible – either to the scientific community or to the general public.

'Exotic' ingredients in cosmetic preparations are usually derived from plants, and less frequently from animal organs or tissues. A general rule that applies to a specific ingredient in any cosmetic preparation is the following:

• As long as there has not been reliable, reproducible (meaning that if the experiment is repeated by other researchers, similar results are obtained) scientific research carried out on the product, its efficacy may not be established.

It is likely that there are many substances that may be useful for skin care and protection, but about which no studies have been published in the accredited medical literature. It is reasonable to assume that there are other natural substances whose potential has not yet been identified, and that will eventually find their way into the cosmetics industry.

What do we know about the active ingredients in cosmetic preparations?
The various active ingredients of cosmetic preparations can be classified into the following categories:

Animal-derived substances
This group includes the various proteins (such as collagen and elastin), various amino acids, nucleic acids, hyaluronic acid, placental extract, amniotic fluid and ceramides.

Plant extracts
This group includes substances obtained from a wide range of plants, such as aloe vera, lavender, camomile, calendula, echinacea, jojoba oil and tea-tree oil. The **aromatic oils** also belong to this group. They are derived from eucalyptus, camphor, mint and jasmine, and also from the camomile and lavender plants. The **phytosterols** include extracts from cocoa butter, coconut, olives, avocado, sesame, sunflower seeds and soya oil. **Gamma-linoleic acid** is derived from the oils of the evening primrose and foxtail plants. **Alpha-hydroxy acids** are derived originally from fruits and vegetables, so they can also be included in this category. They are discussed in detail in Chapter 17. **Allantoin** is included here because in the past it was extracted from various plants, although it is now produced synthetically from uric acid.

Vitamins
These include vitamins C and E, beta-carotene, and provitamin B (pantothenic acid).

Foodstuffs
Many cosmetics in use for centuries in various cultures are based on food-stuffs, such as milk, eggs, honey and propolis.

Naturally occurring substances extracted from animal tissues

Collagen
This protein, in the form of collagen fibers, is a major component of the skin. Many consumers mistakenly believe that the collagen in cosmetic prepara-tions can penetrate the skin and replace the 'old' collagen. This, of course, is incorrect. Because of its high molecular weight, collagen cannot penetrate the keratinous layer of the skin and enter into the 'living' skin layers.

The only way in which collagen can effectively penetrate the skin is by injection into the deep layers of the skin, in order to treat depressed scars or wrinkles. In this case, collagen provides no benefit other than to 'raise' the wrinkles or depressed scars, and even then its effect is only temporary, since the injected collagen becomes absorbed within months.

Note that collagen can increase the moisture content of the skin, since it absorbs water effectively. The feeling of improvement in the skin's appear-ance after applying cosmetic products containing collagen is probably due to this increased moisture in the skin. In addition, collagen may be used in hair-care products, especially those intended for hair that has been damaged by incorrect treatment (see the section on protein conditioners in Chapter 27).

Amino acids, elastin and other proteins

Like collagen, these substances cannot penetrate the keratinous layer of the skin, and do not get into the epidermis. Some of them absorb water, however, so they can have a beneficial effect on the skin by increasing its moisture content. There is no scientific evidence that these substances can delay skin ageing or the appearance of wrinkles.

Nucleic acids

Various combinations of nucleic acids form DNA – the genetic material in all living cells that contains the genetic code. There is no proof that nucleic acids or DNA itself have any effect on preventing skin ageing. These substances do absorb water, and can increase the moisture content of the skin to a certain extent.

Hyaluronic acid

The dermis is largely made up of an amorphous intercellular substance (i.e. a substance that has no defined shape or structure), which serves as 'cement' for all the components of the dermis. One of the substances making up the intercellular material in the dermis is hyaluronic acid, which is an efficient water-absorbing substance. Hyaluronic acid is becoming widely used in moisturizing compounds.

Amniotic fluid

The concept of using amniotic fluid, which surrounds the developing fetus in the womb, has connotations of 'rejuvenation' and prevention of skin ageing. Amniotic fluid used in the cosmetics industry comes from pregnant cows, and is obtained by puncturing the amniotic sac with a needle inserted through the cow's uterus. The beneficial effect of these products has not been proven by scientific experiments.

Placental extracts

As with amniotic fluid the fact that the placenta (the afterbirth) is intimately bound up with fetal development leads some consumers to feel that it influences rejuvenation and prevents ageing of the skin. From a scientific point of view, this has not been proven.

There are cosmetic products containing complex mixtures of various placentally derived enzymes and other proteins, which differ according to the industrial processing of the extracts from animal and human placentas (note that in most countries the use of human tissue for cosmetics is forbidden). This processing involves rinsing the tissues (to remove blood), and then extracting the clean placental tissue.

It appears, however, that this process is now being used less. One possible reason is that placental tissue is particularly well supplied with blood vessels. In recent years the use of any product related to blood has become anathema to consumers because of possible contamination by viral or bacterial diseases. Although the transmission of infectious diseases by placental extracts has never been documented, the market for these products is on the decline.

Ceramides

Ceramides make up approximately 40% of the fatty acids in the cells of the body, and are a significant component of the keratin layer. They are important in protecting its integrity. It has been shown that applying products containing ceramides to the skin of animals creates an impermeable, insulating layer for the outer skin layers. Recently, cosmetics companies have developed ointments containing ceramides in various concentrations – both as moisturizing preparations and as protective substances to prevent and repair skin damage resulting from exposure to various chemicals (including soaps that damage the keratin layer of the skin). Some people attribute to ceramides a certain ability to prevent skin ageing, but this has not yet been proven by scientific testing. Nevertheless, there is no doubt that even if a small part of the potential properties of these substances were realized, they would represent a breakthrough in cosmetic treatment.

Plant extracts

Plant extracts have a wide range of effects. Some provide a pleasant scent or attractive colour to cosmetic preparations; some provide moisture to the skin and act as 'skin softeners' (usually the fattier extracts). Certain extracts are known for their 'soothing' properties (such as camomile or aloe vera extracts), and others, such as witch hazel extract, as astringents (astringents are discussed in detail in Chapter 19).

It should be remembered that not all the extracts derived from a given plant are uniform or identical. There may be subtypes or different varieties of a plant, whose extracts may have quite different pharmacological properties from one another. Sometimes the extracts vary depending on the season of the year during which the plant was picked, and sometimes their pharmacological properties depend on the method of extraction used. In certain cases, the main effect of the final product actually depends on other substances present in the product containing the plant extract.

No extract of any plant has yet been proven scientifically to have an effect on skin ageing or on rejuvenation (apart from what is discussed in Chapter 17 on alpha-hydroxy acids).

Some plant extracts are claimed to have antibacterial or antifungal properties. When dealing with skin that is infected or irritated it is preferable to use accepted medical preparations (after consulting with a physician) rather than plant extracts: conventional medicine has a wide range of dermatological medications that have been proven to be effective against bacteria and fungi, and are known to be safe.

The following pages give details of a number of plant extracts in common use in the cosmetics industry. The discussion here is largely based on accepted, widely known information; but most of the available information is not definite, and further scientific research is needed to verify it.

Aloe vera

Aloe vera is widely used both as a cosmetic and as a home remedy for simple cuts and burns, and for skin irritation. In cosmetics, it is present in every conceivable product: creams, ointments, soaps, shampoos, tanning lotions, cleansing lotions, and others.

The 'soothing' effect of aloe vera is well known to the general public. The aloe vera plant was known for its medicinal properties in antiquity in Mesopotamia and Egypt. The Chinese in ancient times were known to have used it for the relief of abdominal pain (it has a cathartic effect when taken by mouth), the Indians used it for treating urinary problems, and throughout history extracts of this plant have been used for skin treatment. The aloe vera plant has yellow flowers, with fleshy leaves arranged in a rosette pattern (see the illustration below), from which the substance is extracted. There are specific subtypes of the plant, in which the composition of the substance may vary chemically and pharmacologically.

Properties attributed to aloe vera

- **Anti-inflammatory properties** have been attributed to various components of the substance: lectin-like substances, carboxypeptidase, magnesium lactate, and others.
- There is an **antibacterial effect** – perhaps because of the component known as saponin, and perhaps due to other substances.
- There is an ability to **accelerate wound healing**.

The results of various research experiments examining the use of aloe vera compared with conventional treatment for various skin infections and burns have been inconclusive, and at times contradictory. Hence one cannot say unequivocally what the value of the substance really is.

Note: There are different species of aloe vera – so there are differences in the pharmacological effects, depending on the specific subtype. The nature and composition of the substance also vary, depending on the season when the

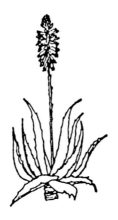

Aloe vera.

plant is picked. Sometimes the other components in the preparation in which the substance is found can change and neutralize the effect of the active ingredient. Different methods of extraction can produce differences in the composition and effects of the extracts. Hence one product containing aloe vera may have a beneficial effect on the skin, while another product may be useless. The major ingredient responsible for the various effects (anti-inflammatory, antibacterial) has not been definitely identified, so that further research is needed to determine the efficacy of the substance and the purposes for which it is best suited.

Lavender

Lavender is extracted from the flowers of *Lavendula officinalis*; the oil derived from it has a pleasant scent. Some claim that the substances extracted from lavender for use on the skin have anti-oxidant properties. Other products are used for soothing skin irritation and inflammation. Lavender is used mainly for producing various fragrances. In addition, an aromatic oil can be extracted from it.

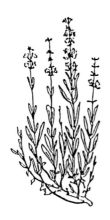

Lavender.

Camomile

Camomile is derived from the flowers of two plants: *Anthemis nobilis*, known as Roman camomile, and *Matricaria chamomilla*, known as German camomile. The extracts from both of these plants have a pleasant fragrance. Drinking camomile extract is said to have soothing effects on the digestive system. Those products derived from the camomile plant for use on the skin are claimed to possess anti-inflammatory effects and to be able to constrict blood vessels – properties that help to soothe skin irritations. Tea made from camomile (after it has cooled down) is used widely in dermatological practice as a mouthwash in cases of painful mouth sores. In addition, a recommended treatment for swelling around the eyes is to place cotton compresses soaked in camomile extract (or cooled camomile tea) on the swollen area for a few minutes several times a day. In a few isolated cases, camomile extract has been found to have a certain effect on the healing of wounds – but this has never been confirmed scientifically.

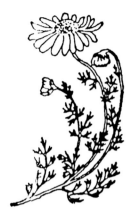

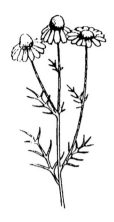

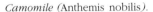

Camomile (Anthemis nobilis).

Camomile (Matricaria chamomilla).

Calendula

The extract derived from the petals of *Calendula officinalis* is said to have anti-inflammatory properties, and is used for the treatment of mild skin irritation. The extract also is said to be a mild astringent. Some have suggested that it also has antibacterial and antifungal properties.

Echinacea

Echinacea is a medicinal herb that grows in North and South America, and has been used for centuries. The extract is usually obtained from the root of the plant. The extract is said to be effective mainly against infections – bacteria, fungi and viruses. This effect is purported to be related to the ability of the extract to neutralize a substance called **hyaluronidase**, which is secreted by bacteria. There have not been any reports in the scientific literature of controlled scientific studies performed on echinacea extract to document this effect. Echinacea has never been proven to be as effective as the antibiotic medications.

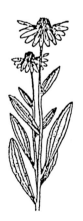

Echinacea.

Hyaluronidase

Hyaluronidase is an enzyme secreted by bacteria. It is able to dissolve and break down **hyaluronic acid**, which, as mentioned earlier in this chapter, is part of the intercellular material in the dermis. The assumption is that by neutralizing and blocking hyaluronidase, echinacea extract prevents possible damage to body tissues caused by bacteria or fungi.

Australian tea-tree oil

The oil of the Australian tea tree (*Melaleuca alternifolia*) is extracted after distilling its leaves. It is a colourless to clear-yellow liquid, which has a characteristic scent that is generally considered to be pleasant. This substance has been used for centuries by Australian aborigines. It is marketed as an antibacterial and antifungal preparation, and does have some antiseptic properties. Tea-tree oil is also said to have a soothing effect on the skin. It is meant to be used on skin inflammations, bacterial or fungal infections, and minor cuts or burns. It appears in several forms – as an emulsion, a cream or an ointment. In a scientific study published in Australia in 1990, the substance was found to have some beneficial effect on acne.

Jojoba oil

Jojoba oil , derived from a plant that grows in Mexico and southwestern North America, is widely used as a folk remedy. Some twenty years ago people began using it as a component in shampoos, hair conditioners and moisturizing creams. In the last decade, it has been introduced into cosmetic and medical preparations. Jojoba oil penetrates the keratinous layer of the skin very well. Several researchers have been able to demonstrate that it reaches the dermis, and attempts have been made to use it as a carrier to deliver other substances deep into the skin. In addition, it has been suggested that jojoba oil can decrease excessive sebaceous gland secretion, and that it has certain beneficial effects on mild skin inflammation and irritation.

Aromatic oils

Aromatic oils have been used for millennia – by the ancient Greeks and in ancient Egypt – for pain relief and as sedatives. These oils, derived from various plants, are volatile liquids with a characteristic fragrance. They may be extracted from different parts of plants – not just from the flowers and fruit, but also from the roots of certain plants and the trunks of some trees. Aromatic oils are reputed to possess anti-inflammatory and antibacterial properties. Some have analgesic (pain relief) properties, and some such as menthol and camphor, have a cooling effect on the skin.

It should be noted that, because of their unique fragrances, some of the aromatic oils affect emotional and psychological processes to some extent, and they can modulate mood and general well-being. This effect may be related to a central mechanism in the brain that is connected to the sense of smell. Some of these substances (e.g. mint oil) have a stimulatory effect, while others (e.g. rose oil and jasmine oil) have a calming, soothing effect.

There is a wide range of uses made of aromatic oils in the cosmetics industry:

- in shampoos, hair conditioners and hair curling preparations;
- in soaps, such as camomile soap, which increases the moisture content of the skin and gives a feeling of 'smooth skin' during and after bathing; similarly, adding aromatic oils in a concentration of about 1% to soaps provides a degree of antibacterial effect;
- in various deodorants, because of their fragrance and the antibacterial effect;
- they are also used in insect repellents.

Recently more and more use is being made of the mood-altering properties of aromatic oils – for relaxation and also for stimulation. Several cosmetics companies produce an 'energizing shampoo' and also a shampoo with a soothing fragrance. The energizing shampoo contains 'stimulatory' oils, such as camphor and mint, whereas a shampoo with a soothing fragrance may contain jasmine or rose oils.

Phytosterols

Phytosterols have a similar chemical structure to cholesterol, and are extracted from various plant sources, such as cocoa butter, coconut, olives, avocados, sesame, sunflower seeds and soya oil. Their major biological effect is anti-inflammatory, and their use in cosmetics is mainly related to this property. Phytosterols are usually present in anti-inflammatory creams for people with dry skin, in sunburn creams, and in creams for the treatment of various inflammatory conditions of the skin, including diaper rash in infants (resulting from skin contact with various irritating substances, such as urine and stool). It is usual to include a mixture of phytosterols, such as avocado oil or similar compounds, in hair care products. These combinations act to condition and soften the hair; the lowering of the electrostatic charge of the hair by these compounds may prevent the 'shapeless' wispy look.

Gamma-linoleic acid

Gamma-linoleic acid is a fatty acid that is said to have anti-inflammatory properties. It also acts as an insulating, impermeable substance in the keratin layer of the skin, thereby improving the skin's protective qualities. In cosmetics, gamma-linoleic acid is used mainly as an ingredient in various moisturizing compounds.

In dermatology, there have been reports of a beneficial effect in the treatment of atopic dermatitis using **evening primrose oil** (which contains a high concentration of gamma-linoleic acid).

Another oil that contains large amounts of gamma-linoleic acid is **borage oil**. The regular application of cosmetics containing borage oil for several weeks or more lessens the amount of moisture lost through the skin. Skin damage with dryness and roughness of the skin, resulting from the frequent use of detergents such as sodium lauryl sulfate (a common ingredient in soaps and shampoos), has been successfully treated by the regular application of preparations containing borage oil.

Allantoin

Allantoin used to be extracted from various plants, but today, in the cosmetics industry, it is made synthetically from uric acid. Allantoin is considered a 'soothing' substance for irritated skin, and it is claimed that it has some effect on the repair of wounds, but there is no scientific substantiation of those claims. Allantoin is a **keratolytic** substance, which means that it is able to soften and dissolve the keratin (horny) layer of the skin, by virtue of its action on the keratin protein that makes up this layer. It is a common ingredient in moisturizing substances and products used to diminish skin irritation. It is used, for example, in treating thickened, dry skin and cracked lips, and it is a common ingredient in shampoos for the treatment of dandruff.

Vitamins

Vitamins, by definition, are organic compounds of various types, present in small amounts in food, and whose presence is essential for the normal physiological function of the body.

The term 'vitamin' holds a special marketing magic in the cosmetics industry, but in fact the beneficial effect of some vitamins on the skin remains unproved. The last decade has seen enormous interest in vitamins with antioxidant properties. These include vitamin C, beta-carotene and vitamin E. The assumption is that these vitamins can trap oxygen free radicals, which cause damage to body tissues. Many research studies have been carried out to determine whether, in fact, the addition of these vitamins to the diet can decrease the incidence of heart disease, blood vessel disease and cancer. Although some studies seemed to support this, the topic is still controversial. Furthermore, the question of whether the addition of these vitamins improves the quality of the skin, and slows down the process of skin ageing, is still undecided.

What are oxygen free radicals?

Oxygen free radicals, byproducts of chemical changes in the oxygen molecule, are continuously being produced in body tissues. The production of oxygen free radicals increases in response to certain situations, such as exposure to the sun and to X-rays, smoking, and environmental pollution.

Oxygen free radicals damage cell walls in the body, damage the genetic material (DNA) in the cells, and may alter various biochemical compounds within cells. It appears that oxygen free radicals play a significant role in heart and blood vessel disease, and in the development of malignancies. Scientists believe that the gradual, cumulative effect of oxygen free radicals accelerates the ageing process in the various body systems (including the skin). Also, solar skin damage is largely thought to be due to the effect of oxygen free radicals.

What do we know about the use of these vitamins when applied to the skin?

Until recently, the classic argument of those who denied the effectiveness of products containing these vitamins when applied to the skin was that the vitamins are unable to penetrate the keratinous layer of the skin, and hence cannot reach the epidermis or dermis. However, recent scientific research has shown that vitamins C and E, when present in some skin preparations, do in fact penetrate the epidermis, and are absorbed. Their degree of penetration depends on their concentration, and on the composition of the other substances in the preparation. It should be remembered, however, that although these vitamins can penetrate the epidermis and dermis, this still does not mean that they necessarily have any beneficial effect on the skin, or that they act as anti-oxidants and trap oxygen free radicals, and in that way improve the quality of the skin.

Vitamin C

The assumption is that vitamin C, in skin preparations, has anti-oxidant properties that protect the skin from damage caused by ultraviolet radiation, air pollution and smoke. Furthermore, vitamin C plays a role in stimulating cells in the dermis to produce collagen, so that applying skin preparations containing this vitamin may be of some value.

Note: It must be emphasized that when we talk of vitamin C's function in protecting the skin from the sun and ultraviolet radiation, we are not implying that it is acting as a screen that filters out or reflects the damaging rays. What we mean is that apparently it has some effect on the repair of pre-existing sun and radiation damage.

Vitamin A

In the standard scientific literature there is no proof that topical preparations containing vitamin A have any beneficial effect on the skin. On the other hand, retinoic acid, a compound similar in chemical structure to vitamin A, has been proven to have a beneficial effect on the skin. Retinoic acid and its effects are discussed in detail in Chapter 16.

Provitamin B (panthenol)

This substance is claimed to be able to aid in the healing of wounds and to lessen skin inflammation. It is therefore a common ingredient of products designed for treating diaper rash in infants.

Vitamins: in summary

So far, there have been no controlled scientific studies on humans published that have unequivocally confirmed that skin preparations containing vitamins have a beneficial effect on the skin. Nevertheless, more and more evidence is starting to accumulate that suggests that they may do so. Further research is needed to verify that vitamins in cosmetic products benefit the skin.

Common foodstuffs

Eggs and milk

Apart from their nutritional value, there is no evidence that cosmetic preparations containing eggs or milk have anything to contribute to skin care, other than perhaps improving the moisture content of the skin and thereby imparting a smooth texture to it. Even if they do, the same results can be obtained from standard moisturizing substances.

Honey, propolis and Royal bee jelly

These substances have been in use for many years in folk medicine – mainly for healing wounds. Honey has been found to have certain properties in the treatment of burns. This effect, it is presumed, is related to the high concentration of sugars in honey, which prevents the growth of bacteria on the injury. Nevertheless, with regard to the healing of burns, honey has never been proven to be as effective as the standard antibacterial substances used in these cases. No other beneficial effect of honey or propolis on the skin (such as prevention of skin ageing) has been proven.

Some additional comments

The meaning of the word 'natural' in cosmetics

We stress that not everything that has the label 'natural' should automatically be used or recommended. Indeed, various medications used for treating serious diseases are manufactured by a completely synthetic process. And without doubt, treatment with these 'synthetic' substances is by far preferable to the course (totally natural) of illness, or of death. Thus, by the same token, for example, a baby hair shampoo made of a synthetic substance is generally less harmful and less irritating to the skin than is normal soap, which is derived from 'natural' animal fats. Not only that, but not all preparations marketed as 'natural', are indeed such. In the course of the manufacture of so-called 'natural' products, there is usually a whole chain of processes – sterilization, alcohol disinfection, and the addition of preservatives, artificial colouring agents and fragrances. As the product reaches the consumer it is usually totally different from its natural, basic form; although it too, may be marketed as 'natural'.

It is certainly advisable to avoid adding synthetic substances to a cosmetic product. It is also advisable to avoid unnecessary processing steps in the manufacture of cosmetics. Nevertheless, the label 'natural' should be viewed with circumspection. More important than the degree of 'naturalness' of a product are factors such as the following: What is known about its side-effects? How irritating or damaging to the skin is the substance? To what extent has its efficacy been proven?

Preparations purporting to 'enrich the skin with oxygen'

Some cosmetic preparations are advertised as 'providing oxygen to the skin'. However, it should be remembered that the skin receives its oxygen through blood vessels in the dermis, and, provided there is no damage to that blood supply, the skin needs no alternative source of oxygen. Not only that – today considerable research is being devoted to the question of possible damage caused by oxygen and its byproducts (free oxygen radicals) to various tissues, including the skin. Indeed, there are products (such as vitamin E) that are used specifically because of their anti-oxidant effects (see above).

The concept of 'skin nutrition'

When a cosmetic product is said to 'nourish the skin', this usually means that it contains ingredients that have a biological effect on skin cells. All the substances covered in this chapter come into this category – some have scientific 'backing' for their biological activity, while others have no scientific proof of their beneficial value or their biological effect on the skin. In general, the skin (epidermis and dermis) obtains its nutrients via the blood vessels in the skin, and not from substances applied to its surface. Preparations said to 'nourish the skin' are generally fatty substances that are relatively impermeable to water. They are usually applied at night, and are meant to remain on the skin for several hours. They contain various active ingredients supposed to benefit the skin after penetrating deeply. Remember that in terms of 'nutrition', cells and tissues do not take up substances in their original forms. Proteins are broken down in the digestive system to amino acids, which are then absorbed into the bloodstream; fats are broken down to fatty acid units; most sugars are broken down to single-sugar units. Thus, the body tissues, including the skin, are neither 'used to' nor able to take up complex molecules such as proteins.

Penetration of substances into the skin cells

The cell membrane represents the outer surface of the cell. It acts as a selective barrier that regulates the entry and exit of substances in and out of the cell. The cell membrane is made up of phospholipids (fatty compounds containing phosphorus), proteins and polysaccharides (complex sugars).

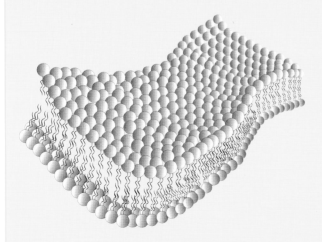

Microscopic structure of the cell membrane, made up of a double layer of phospholipids.

As can be seen in the illustration, the phospholipids are organized in a double layer. This arrangement of the cell wall prevents the unwanted passage of fatty substances or water-soluble substances in or out of the cell.

Liposomes were developed in order to allow the penetration of substances into the epidermis and dermis, and thence into the skin cells. The logic behind the development of liposomes is that, just like the cell wall, they are made of phospholipids. The assumption is that they will therefore be able to become attached to the cell wall and penetrate it.

The use of liposomes enables various active ingredients to penetrate the keratin layer of the skin, which is made up of closely packed layers of cells. This is discussed in detail in Chapter 21.

Note that recently cosmetic preparations containing various vitamins, particularly vitamins C and E, have been developed. It is possible that a certain level of these vitamins can get to the cells of the epidermis and dermis, so one could regard this as a certain form of 'skin nourishment'.

16
Retinoic acid

Contents Overview • The beneficial effects • Who may benefit from retinoic acid? • Guidelines for use • Side-effects • Warnings • Conclusion

Overview

An important turning point in the world of cosmetic dermatology occurred with the development of retinoic acid, a synthetic retinoid compound. Retinoids resemble vitamin A in their chemical composition and are used in the treatment of several skin diseases.

The regular application of products containing retinoic acid improves, to a certain extent, the signs of **photoageing** (skin damaged by exposure to the sun) and **chronological skin ageing**, related to increasing age.

Retinoic acid was originally intended for acne treatment. Dermatologists observed its beneficial effect on the skin when treating adult women with acne. These patients reported that their skin became somewhat smoother, and fine wrinkles flattened and nearly disappeared. Dark facial blemishes were lightened, and some even vanished.

Subsequently, the efficacy of the product was compared with creams with similar ingredients but without retinoic acid. These creams were applied for prolonged periods, each on a different side of the face. The studies proved the efficacy of retinoic acid, both in the prevention of skin ageing and in improving pre-existing damage.

The beneficial effects

Retinoic acid lessens the consequences of photoageing. In addition, there is some beneficial effect of retinoic acid on chronological skin ageing, which appears with the passage of time.

- At the microscopic level, retinoic acid enhances cell division in the **epidermis**, replacing damaged and unorganized cells with new organized cells. It also reduces melanin production. In the **dermis**, new collagen and elastic fibres are formed.

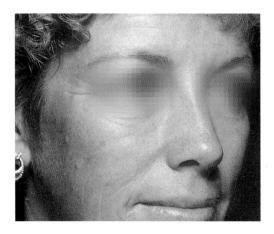

(a) Wrinkles before treatment.

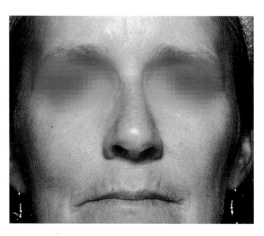

(a) Before treatment.

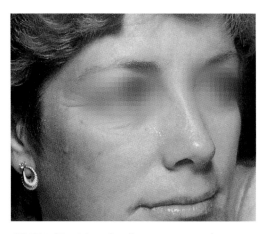

(b) Wrinkles 24 weeks after treatment with retinoic acid.

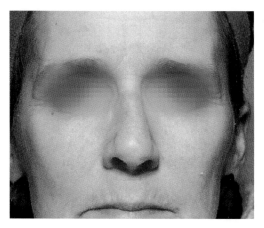

(b) 24 weeks after treatment with retinoic acid.

- The skin becomes visibly smoother and thicker. Retinoic acid can cause significant flattening and diminishing, and even disappearance, of fine wrinkles in the skin.
- Dark blemishes on the face (brownish-yellow or light-brown lesions, often referred to as **age spots** or **liver spots**), can lighten and sometimes disappear. (The precise medical term for 'age spots' is **solar lentigines**, which are also referred to as **senile lentigines**. Further details are provided in Chapter 18 on bleaching preparations.)
- Regular application of retinoic acid may cause the regression or disappearance of precancerous lesions such as **solar keratoses**, although this is not necessarily the sole or preferred treatment for such lesions. The treatment of solar keratoses should only be carried out by a physician.
- Retinoic acid increases the blood flow in the skin, producing a pinkish 'healthy' colour.

The beneficial effect of treatment with retinoic acid is gradual and prolonged, and significant improvement may be apparent only after several months. Maximal improvement occurs within the first year of treatment. In the first year, the ageing process is delayed, and even somewhat reversed. If treatment is continued for more than a year, the delaying effect continues, but further repair of already-damaged skin cannot be expected.

Prolonged, severe damage caused by the sun cannot be fully corrected. Nevertheless, many patients are pleased with the results. Expectations should be realistic. The product is not a substitute for relatively aggressive treatments, such as chemical peeling of the skin or surgical intervention. Neither deep wrinkles nor expression lines can be corrected by such treatment – the results are apparent only on fine wrinkles. Nor will all dark facial blemishes be lightened by the product, so alternative regimens should be considered for certain types of skin lesions.

Note: The labels of many cosmetic products contain the names of compounds that are chemically similar to retinoic acid, such as retinol, pro-retinol, retinaldehyde, etc. The fact that these compounds can be sold without a doctor's prescription allows them to be marketed freely.

Some dermatologists agree that prolonged use of retinol or retinaldehyde may have beneficial effects on the skin, similar (but weaker) to that of retinoic acid. However, one should keep in mind that whilst the beneficial effect of retinoic acid is documented in many research studies, retinol or retinaldehyde have been less well studied with respect to their potential effect on the process of skin ageing and photoageing.

Who may benefit from retinoic acid?

Retinoic acid is primarily beneficial for individuals over the age of 35 years with evidence of photoageing – lesions caused by excessive sun exposure. These are manifested by the appearance of fine wrinkles and dark blemishes. Patients with skin damage due to chronological ageing also benefit from treatment with retinoic acid.

Mechanism of action of topical retinoic acid

Initially retinoic acid binds to a specific protein found within cells of the skin. This protein (**cellular retinoic acid binding protein**) transports retinoic acid into the nucleus of each cell. The next stage is within the nucleus. By binding to specific nuclear proteins, retinoic acid modulates the expression of genes, thus altering the processes of growth and maturation of the cells in the epidermis and the dermis.

Guidelines for use

Retinoic acid is a drug. Therefore it must be purchased with a physician's prescription, and precise directions must be followed, under the supervision of a physician. The treatment is individually prescribed by the physician, determined according to age, skin type, history of sun exposure and possible sensitivities to specific medications.

Retinoic acid is marketed in three concentrations:

- 0.025%
- 0.05%
- 0.1%

Treatment should be initiated with the lowest available concentration, and this should be increased gradually, as necessary. The product is usually applied as a cream, but in the case of very oily skin a gel may be favoured. The face should be washed with a gentle soap prior to the application of retinoic acid. The product should be applied at night, and washed away in the morning, since it increases sensitivity to the sun. The product should be applied to the:

- face
- upper chest
- outer arms
- backs of the hands

A very small amount should be applied. Dermatologists state that a very small quantity (a pea-sized amount) should suffice for an area of skin the size of the forehead.

At first, retinoic acid should be applied nightly. For sensitive skin, application should be started with once every other night, and gradually increased to nightly application. After one year, when maximal improvement has been attained and the condition of the skin has stabilized, application of the product two or three times weekly may be sufficient for continued preventive treatment.

During treatment, activities that damage skin, such as sun exposure or smoking, should be avoided. In the daytime, the face should be protected with appropriate sunscreen and moisturizers. The purpose of moisturizers is to avoid dryness of the face, resulting from the application of retinoic acid. Retinoic acid should not be applied at the same time as moisturizers, since this combination may cause adverse effects.

Side-effects

When first applied, retinoic acid reduces the thickness of the outer epidermal layer as well as the horny layer, which retains skin moisture. Only at a later stage does the product affect cell division in the epidermis and cause epidermal thickening. Consequently, most patients will initially notice a dry sensation with slight scaling. This occurs within two weeks to three months of the beginning of treatment. Therefore a cream-based product is preferable to a gel-based one, since gel tends to dry skin to a greater extent. The gel form is recommended only for oily skin. If necessary, moisturizing cream should be applied to the face during the day.

Within two weeks of the beginning of treatment, the skin may become irritated. This irritation is manifested by redness and a slight stinging, which disappears within two to three months. This is a well-documented effect, and if it is not extreme, treatment may be continued.

When redness or stinging is especially irritating, a physician should be consulted. The following should be considered:

- discontinue application for several days
- decrease the concentration of active product
- decrease the amount of cream or gel
- use every second or third day, when renewing application

Note: the burning sensation and the therapeutic effect are probably not related. Slight stinging in the treated region is normal, and can be anticipated. However, any patient with a reaction that is more severe than slight stinging should follow the guidelines above.

Warnings

Avoid sun exposure when using retinoic acid
Retinoic acid increases sensitivity to the sun, so application must be at night, and the face should be washed in the morning. The product should not be applied during the day, and sun exposure should be avoided. A moisturizer should be applied during the day, with an adequate sunscreen.

Obviously, there is no point in treating sun-damaged skin while at the same time exposing the skin to the harmful rays of the sun.

Avoid combining retinoic acid with other cosmetic products at the same time
Retinoic acid should not be applied at the same time as other cosmetic products. It is not stable when combined with other products. However, it is possible, and quite acceptable practice, to combine the use of retinoic acid preparations with other cosmetic products – but not at the same time. For example, a sunscreen may be used in the morning while retinoic acid is intended for nighttime use. By the same token, retinoic acid preparations may be combined with antibacterial preparations to increase the efficacy of treatment of acne.

In any case, it is best to avoid concomitant use of retinoic acid with cosmetics that may cause skin irritation, such as astringents and 'strong' soaps.

Retinoic acid should not be used during pregnancy
Oral retinoids have a **teratogenic effect**, causing birth defects in the fetus. Although no such defects have been documented following use of a cream

containing retinoic acid, dermatologists do not recommend the use of topical retinoic acid during pregnancy.

Avoid physical contact with eyes or mouth

A small amount of the product can be applied near the lower eyelids or lips. A certain beneficial effect is produced by applying around the mouth and at the outer edges of the eyes. Nevertheless, it is best to be cautious and avoid direct contact of the product with eyes or mouth.

Avoid combining retinoic acid with certain medications

Topical retinoic acid can be combined with most medications. However, it is best not to combine it with medications that may increase the skin's sensitivity to the sun. A dermatologist should be consulted in any case of oral drug ingestion concomitant with the use of topical retinoic acid.

Conclusion

Despite the warnings given above – which must be observed – retinoic acid has a beneficial effect. It appears to delay the ageing process of the skin, and even reverses it to a certain extent.

17

Alpha-hydroxy acids

Contents Overview • Effects of low concentrations of alpha-hydroxy acids • Effects of moderate concentrations (up to 50%) of alpha-hydroxy acids on sun-damaged skin • High concentrations of alpha-hydroxy acids for superficial chemical peeling • Guidelines for use • Possible side-effects • Summary

Overview

Alpha-hydroxy acids are a group of compounds derived from various plant sources:

- **glycolic acid**, derived from sugar cane
- **malic acid**, derived from apples
- **tartaric acid**, derived from grapes
- **citric acid**, derived from lemons

Lactic acid, which also belongs to this group, is derived from sour milk. Because most of these acids are of plant origin, they are also known as 'fruit acids' or 'natural acids'. However, most of the alpha-hydroxy acids used in cosmetics are manufactured in laboratories by industrial methods.

Reports in recent years have suggested that preparations containing alpha-hydroxy acids may have a beneficial role to play in skin ageing processes – particularly in those ageing processes related to excessive sun exposure.

The first reports of their use go back a long way. Cleopatra was said to have bathed in milk, which contains lactic acid (although to the best of our knowledge she did not document its effect scientifically). It was a researcher named van Scott and his colleagues from Philadelphia who reintroduced the use of these substances; they recognized the beneficial effects of alpha-hydroxy acids and published a series of scientific articles on the subject.

Of the alpha-hydroxy acids, glycolic acid is the most widely used. Nevertheless, some manufacturers produce alpha-hydroxy products based on lactic acid, citric acid , and other acids, or combinations of these with glycolic acid.

Alpha-hydroxy acids are used in a wide range of preparations, such as:

- creams
- liquid emulsions

- ointments
- gels
- cleansing agents

(In general, alpha-hydroxy acids are less efficient when they are incorporated in cleansing agents than when thay are included in other cosmetic preparations, since in the former case they will be in contact with the skin for a short time only.)

The higher the concentration of the alpha-hydroxy acid, the more marked its effects on the skin. The various preparations can therefore be divided into three groups on the basis of their concentrations of alpha-hydroxy acid:

- **Low concentrations – up to 10%:** These are preparations that can be bought freely over the counter at cosmetics departments. The concentration of alpha-hydroxy acid in preparations that may be sold freely, without a physician's supervision, varies from country to country, and within countries, in accordance with the regulations of the local licensing authorities.
- **Concentrations up to 50%:** These preparations, which require a physician's supervision, are used for a very superficial chemical peeling of the skin. They are usually used in a series of treatments; the treatment is repeated every few days.
- **Concentrations from 50% to 70%:** Alpha-hydroxy acids in these concentrations are used by physicians to achieve superficial chemical peeling of the skin.

In general, the effect of alpha-hydroxy acids depends mainly on their concentration, as well as on the length of time they are in contact with the skin, and the frequency of application. As stated above, the higher the concentration, the more effective the treatment – but then there is more likelihood of skin irritation and undesirable side-effects.

Effects of low concentrations of alpha-hydroxy acids

- At low concentrations (up to 10%), glycolic acid weakens the bonds between the degenerating and dead cells of the outer layers of the skin, thus weakening their adhesion to each other. Hence the keratinous layer cannot build up, and the new cells coming up from below replace the cells that peel away. The replacement of the dry, damaged keratinous layer by a new, thinner, keratinous layer gives the skin a smooth, 'young' appearance.
- Glycolic acid acts as a humectant (absorbs water). Thus, in effect, it functions as a moisturizing cream, resulting in swelling of the skin, with the consequent disappearance of fine wrinkles: dry, rough skin becomes smoother and softer. Therefore the immediate improvement in the appearance of dry skin after applying an alpha-hydroxy acid is mostly attributed to the improvement in the skin's moisture content.

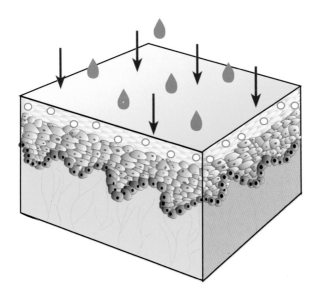

Alpha-hydroxy acids (shown as clear circles) act as water-absorbing particles in the keratin layer.

Note that the effect of alpha-hydroxy acids as moisturizing agents is more prolonged than that of the standard moisturizing agents. The effect of the latter lasts for a few hours, while the beneficial effects of alpha-hydroxy acids may even last for several days after discontinuing treatment.

• Some alpha-hydroxy acids have anti-inflammatory properties by virtue of being anti-oxidants (preventing possible damage from oxygen free radicals).
• Recently, preliminary articles have appeared in the medical literature confirming that, even at relatively low concentrations, the daily application of alpha-hydroxy acids has a beneficial effect on sun-damaged skin. Alpha-hydroxy acids will lighten dark, hyperpigmented blotches on the skin. There is also improvement and a decrease in the appearance of fine skin wrinkles.
• Preparations of alpha-hydroxy acids in low concentrations have a beneficial effect on acne (see Chapter 9).

Effects of moderate concentrations (up to 50%) of alpha-hydroxy acids on sun-damaged skin

Effects on the epidermis

After applying 25% glycolic acid daily for several months to sun-damaged skin, microscopic examination of the skin shows that the epidermis becomes somewhat thicker, with improvements in texture and general structure; the cells appear more uniform and orderly. The visible effect of this on the skin externally is to make it smoother, with less wrinkles. Since most skin wrinkles appear with increasing age and are the result of prolonged exposure to the sun, related to the accumulation of melanin pigment in the epidermal cells, the renewal and organization of the cell turnover in the epidermis should also lessen the number of wrinkles and improve the skin's appearance. Indeed, many preparations used for bleaching areas of skin contain alpha-hydroxy acids together with other active ingredients.

Effects on the dermis

Researchers have formed the impression that constant use of alpha-hydroxy acids in moderately high concentrations has a beneficial effect on the elastic fibres in the skin, and also results in an increase in the amount of collagen fibres in the skin. Some researchers believe that the alpha-hydroxy acids actually penetrate the dermis and encourage the formation of new collagen fibres.

The 'Minipeel' method

In the USA, cosmeticians are allowed to use products with a concentration of alpha-hydroxy acids of up to 30% for very superficial skin peeling. This technique is called the 'Minipeel' method. The preparation is applied to the face and neck for 30 minutes, once or twice a week.

There are several crucial points in using this treatment:

- It is essential that the face be thoroughly cleaned beforehand to remove traces of oil, dead cells, and dirt. If this is not done, the acid will not penetrate the skin evenly and effectively, but will be absorbed by the oily layer and by the dirt on the skin. The way in which the cleansing is carried out has a significant effect on the final result of the treatment. There are ready-made commercial preparations on the market that are combinations of alpha-hydroxy acids with a cleansing agent.
- Peeling requires that a thin, **even** layer of the substance be applied.
- The preparation must be washed off the face at the time specified in the instructions: **it must not be left on the skin for longer than the specified period**. It should be rinsed off with water or a weak solution of sodium bicarbonate (baking soda).

Note: There is a certain risk of burning the patient's skin using the 'Minipeel' method. Other things can also go wrong, whether related to faulty manufacture of the preparation, or to the individual sensitivity of the patient to one of its ingredients.

In most cases, using moderate concentrations (up to 50%) of alpha-hydroxy acids for facial treatments or 'peeling', does improve the skin texture. However, the reaction to these treatments, and the degree of improvement achieved, may vary considerably from one person to another (even when using identical concentrations of the active substance). It should be remembered that treatment with 50% glycolic acid is safe if carried out

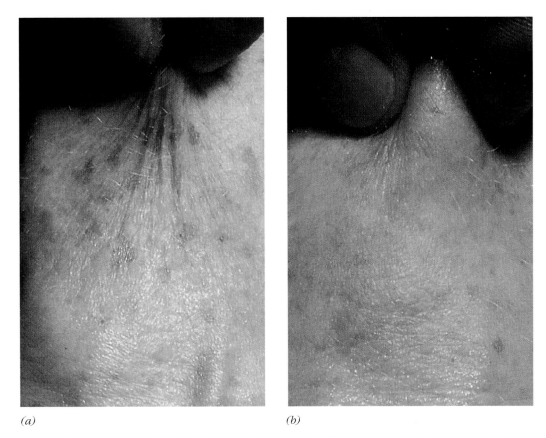

(a)   *(b)*

(a) Right forearm untreated. (b) Left forearm of same patient following six months of treatment with alpha-hydroxy acids (25%). The treated skin is plumper than that of the right forearm, less wrinkled, and with even pigmentation.

by an experienced physician. It is therefore logical to start treatment with this substance first, since, although other products (such as those containing a higher concentration of alpha-hydroxy acid, or other products used for deeper peeling of the skin) may be more effective, they have more side-effects.

High concentrations of alpha-hydroxy acids for superficial chemical peeling

Higher concentrations of alpha-hydroxy acids have a raised acidity level and can burn the skin. Therefore any use of high concentrations of alpha-hydroxy acids requires medical supervision. These highly concentrated solutions (50–70%) are used by physicians to achieve superficial chemical

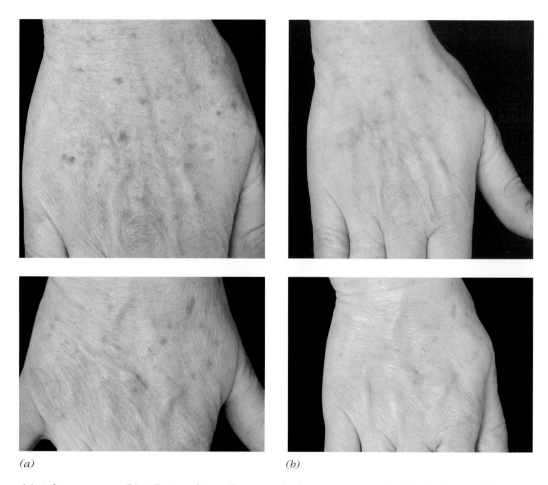

(a) *(b)*

(a) Before treatment. (b) Following skin peeling using high concentrations of alpha-hydroxy acids. The patient was treated with twice-daily applications of glycolic acid 10% lotion and weekly glycolic acid 50% chemical peels for 8 weeks.

peeling of the skin. Chemical peeling of the skin in fact involves 'dissolving' the outer layer of the epidermis. The idea is that after removing this outer layer, new, 'young', healthy skin will grow out to take its place. The effect of the high-concentration preparations depends on the length of time the substance is in contact with the skin, and on the frequency of its use.

Epidermis
After repeated treatment by 70% glycolic acid, on several occasions over a period of months, improvement becomes noticeable in the epidermis. Microscopic examination shows that the epidermis is thicker, while externally the skin looks smoother and slightly thicker, and there are fewer wrinkles.

Dermis

Several research studies on the effects of high concentrations of alpha-hydroxy acids on the skin have suggested that there is formation of new collagen and elastic fibres deep in the dermis.

The main use for deep chemical peeling of the skin using high concentrations of glycolic acid is, as we have stated, for treating sun-damaged skin. In addition, this treatment affords an extra benefit, in that it lightens hyperpigmented (dark) blotches on the skin.

Guidelines for use

Start with low concentrations

The standard recommended technique is to start off with the daily application of an alpha-hydroxy compound with a low concentration of acid (3–4%) to the skin of the face and neck. The treatment is carried out once daily. After a few days it can be applied twice daily, provided that no skin irritation has appeared. Following several weeks of this treatment (again provided that there are no unwanted side-effects), higher concentrations – up to 10% – may be used. Individuals known to have sensitive skin should undergo a skin test of a small area of unexposed skin before using a preparation containing an alpha-hydroxy acid on the entire face.

Alpha-hydroxy compounds in which the concentration of the acid exceeds 10% may only be prescribed by a physician

Sometimes a dermatologist will start treatment in his/her clinic using high concentrations, and then later revert to home treatment with lower concentrations. As noted above, the exact concentration of alpha-hydroxy acid in preparations that may be sold without a physician's supervision varies from country to country, and within countries, in accordance with the regulations of the local licensing authorities.

Prevention of sun exposure

There have recently been reports in the medical literature showing that prolonged use of these compounds can sensitize the skin to ultraviolet radiation. Therefore patients being treated with alpha-hydroxy acids should avoid excessive exposure to sunlight to prevent further skin damage. Patients being treated with these preparations should use a sunscreen with a protective factor appropriate to their degree of sun exposure. Even if the alpha-hydroxy compound is applied in the evening or at night, the patient should still use a sunscreen during the day. In general, it is absurd to use a preparation that prevents and repairs solar skin damage while at the same time exposing oneself to the sun! Note that many preparations containing alpha-hydroxy acids also contain sunscreens.

Combination with retinoic acid

Alpha-hydroxy compounds can be combined with retinoic acid – the alpha-hydroxy compound is applied during the day and the retinoic acid at night.

Some researchers feel that this combination is more effective, and may reduce the effects of ageing on the skin.

Bleaching hyperpigmented lesions

Alpha-hydroxy compounds can be combined with other substances in the treatment of hyperpigmented skin lesions This is discussed in more detail in Chapter 18 on bleaching.

Matching the preparation to the patient's skin type

There is a wide range of alpha-hydroxy compounds to suit a variety of skin types. The product used should be appropriate for the patient's skin type. For example, for a patient with relatively dry facial skin, an oilier preparation should be selected, while for a patient with an oily skin, a gel-based preparation is to be preferred.

Note: There are hundreds of companies manufacturing alpha-hydroxy preparations, with concentrations ranging from 1% to 30%. It must be stressed that the efficacy of an alpha-hydroxy compound depends on how it was prepared, and the constitution of the vehicle in which the acid is dissolved. A glycolic acid cream made by a neighbourhood pharmacist or by a local manufacturing plant may be less effective than one produced by a manufacturer with extensive experience in the manufacture of alpha-hydroxy compounds. Therefore, in general, it is preferable to use products of reputable manufacturers, experienced in the manufacture of alpha-hydroxy compounds.

Possible side-effects

Low concentrations of alpha-hydroxy acids

Stinging, redness, or itching following the application of alpha-hydroxy acids is not common, but can occur. If it does, it usually means that there is excessive sensitivity to one of the components of the product (which can happen with any medical cosmetic product). In that case, one should discontinue applying the preparation. The FDA 1999 instructions regarding alpha-hydroxy acids state that even mild irritation is a sign that the product is causing damage. It is recommended not to use another alpha-hydroxy acid preparation without first consulting a dermatologist.

Moderate or high concentrations of alpha-hydroxy acids

The side-effects can vary in severity: slight irritation will be manifested by redness and stinging. Severe cases associated with higher concentrations may be manifested by the appearance of blistering and painful burns. In these cases, a dermatologist should be consulted.

Restrictions on the use of alpha-hydroxy acids in the USA

The concentration of alpha-hydroxy acid that may be sold freely, without a doctor's prescription, varies, depending on the local licensing authority. In the USA, the Cosmetic Ingredient Review Panel (the cosmetics industry's self-regulatory body for examining the safety of cosmetic ingredients) determined in 1997 that alpha-hydroxy acids are safe to use in cosmetic preparations in concentrations up to 10%, provided that the pH of the preparation is not less than 3.5 (this is because the more acidic the preparation (the lower the pH), the higher the absorption of the alpha-hydroxy acid into the skin).

In the USA, preparations containing up to 30% alpha-hydroxy acid are permitted for use by trained cosmetologists, on condition that the substance is applied to the skin for only brief periods of time, and is then immediately rinsed off. However, in recent years, there have been reports of side-effects from products containing alpha-hydroxy acids. Such reports are more common in cases where the concentration of the alpha-hydroxy acid in the preparation is moderately high, up to 30% – a concentration that, in the USA, may be used by trained cosmetologists. In view of those findings, the current permits and safety regulations in the USA are being re-examined by the Food and Drug Authority (FDA).

Use of alpha-hydroxy acids on dark-skinned patients

The use of alpha-hydroxy preparations on people of Asiatic origin, and dark-skinned people in general, requires particular care (compared with their use in Caucasians). In those people, there is an increased tendency to side-effects such as skin irritation, as well as the appearance of dark (pigmented) skin blotches in the treated areas (post-inflammatory pigmentation). These effects are extremely uncommon following the use of cosmetic preparations sold without a prescription, in which there is a low concentration of the active ingredient. On the other hand, in those preparations used by physicians for peeling, and in which there is a higher concentration of glycolic acid (over 20%), these effects are more common.

In spite of all the above, glycolic acid is considered a very safe substance for achieving skin peeling in dark-skinned people.

Summary

Alpha-hydroxy compounds have a beneficial effect on sun-damaged skin. The only substances shown to have a beneficial effect in lessening the effects of ageing on the skin are alpha-hydroxy acids and retinoic acid.

18

Bleaching and bleaching preparations

Contents Overview: skin colour and melanin • Which skin lesions are bleaching preparations used for? • General remarks regarding bleaching preparations • Bleaching preparations • Other preparations used for bleaching hyperpigmented blotches • Other forms of treatment that can be performed by a physician • Summary

Overview: skin colour and melanin

Skin colour is determined by several factors, the main ones being:

- the **thickness** of the skin;
- the **blood vessels** in the skin: their density and the extent to which they are dilated (the more closely packed and the more dilated the blood vessels are, the redder the skin looks);
- the amount of **oxygen in the blood:** a high level of oxygen in the blood makes the skin bright red, while a low level of oxygen gives the skin a bluish colouration;
- the presence of **pigments** that may alter skin colour: for example, carotene, a substance with a similar chemical structure to vitamin A, gives the skin a yellow tinge – a person who eats an excessive amount of carrots (which contain carotene) will develop a yellowish skin colour typical of carotene accumulation;
- the level of **melanin** in the skin.

Of all the above factors, the most significant is melanin, which is produced by special cells in the skin, called **melanocytes**. The amount of melanin produced depends on several factors:

- race (dark-skinned people produce more melanin)
- genetic factors (heredity)
- hormonal factors
- exposure to the sun

Tanning

The production of melanin following exposure to the sun is manifested by **tan-ning**. To some extent, tanning is a protective mechanism, since melanin provides the skin with natural protection against solar damage. When its level in the skin rises, there is better protection from the sun's rays. However, the protection afford-ed the skin by melanin is inadequate, particularly for fair-skinned people, and repeated exposure to the sun will lead to damage. Some of the damage appears in the form of dark areas on the skin, of varying shades of brown. For further details, see Chapter 10 on sun and the skin.

Many cosmetic problems appear as dark blotches and lesions on the skin, or as uneven distribution of colour throughout the skin. The main reason for these problems is the abnormal and non-uniform distribution of melanin in the skin. A **hypopigmented** lesion is an area of skin in which the amount of melanin is reduced, while a **hyperpigmented** lesion is an area of skin in which the amount of melanin is increased. This chapter discusses problems of hyper-pigmentation – skin lesions that are dark-coloured, and methods of bleaching them.

Note: The treatment of dark (hyperpigmented) skin blotches and lesions must only be performed by a physician.

- Sometimes a hyperpigmented lesion is actually a cancer of the skin. Obvi-ously, the treatment then is not merely to bleach the lesion; such a lesion should be removed and examined microscopically. In any case of a dark lesion, the possibility of melanoma should only be ruled out by a physician.
- There are many preparations for bleaching skin lesions, and it is important that the appropriate and specific preparation be used for each patient, according to his/her medical background.

This chapter is included in the book because dark, hyperpigmented lesions are common. The reader should be familiar with the range of treatments available. However, in this case, the treatment must be carried out only under a physician's instructions.

Which skin lesions are bleaching preparations used for?

Freckles
Freckles are those familiar pale-brown spots, usually found in light-skinned people, with light hair, or in redheads. They are generally small – about 5 mm in diameter. Freckles appear in early childhood, between the ages of two and four years. They commonly occur in areas of skin exposed to the sun: the face (mainly on the nose), the shoulders and the upper back. In the summer, freck-les tend to become darker, while in the winter they tend to become smaller and lighter and may almost disappear.

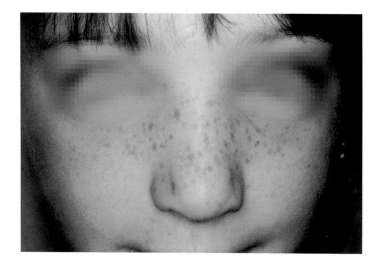

Freckles.

The way to prevent freckles is to avoid excessive exposure to the sun. Some bleaching preparations can bleach freckles to some extent, but these preparations are only partially effective, and will not necessarily make the freckles disappear completely.

'Sun spots'

The correct scientific name for these patches is **solar lentigines**. Some people call them 'liver spots', or 'old-age spots' – unjustifiably, since the main cause of these lesions is repeated exposure to the sun (and so they appear on exposed areas of the body: the face, the backs of the hands, the upper chest and the sides of the arms). They are dark spots, ranging from brown to brown–black. They are usually round or oval, but can be other shapes. 'Sun

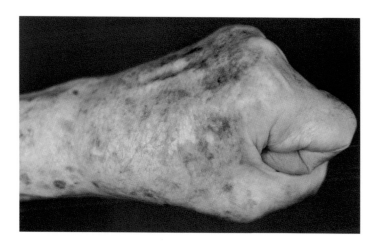

'Sun spots' on the back of the hand.

spots' usually start to appear after the age of 40. They vary in size from a few millimetres to one centimetre. Sometimes a few spots coalesce, forming a larger lesion. This process usually occurs in skin that has been severely damaged as a result of prolonged exposure to the sun over a number of years. 'Sun spots' are discussed further in Chapter 8 on skin ageing and Chapter 10 on sun and the skin, and their treatment is discussed again at the end of the present chapter.

Usually, 'sun spots' pose no danger to health, but are an aesthetic nuisance that most people would prefer to avoid. Minimizing sun exposure will prevent the occurrence of 'sun spots' – or at least diminish the extent of the problem.

Melasma (chloasma, 'pregnancy mask')

Melasma is a unique pattern of pigment distribution on the face. It appears mainly in pregnant women, and is often called a 'pregnancy mask'. In general, there is some accentuation of relatively dark areas of the skin during pregnancy. In its mild form, this phenomenon appears as a darkening of the areola (the area around the nipples). In its more severe form, with involvement of the face, it is called melasma (or chloasma).

Melasma is characterized by the appearance of light to dark brown areas of skin on the face, usually symmetrically distributed. It usually occurs on the upper lip, forehead and chin. It appears as a result of a hormonal process that is not yet understood.

Although melasma appears mainly during pregnancy, it can also occur in women following the use of contraceptives, or of certain hormonal or other medications. Sometimes melasma becomes more prominent before the menstrual period. In many women, it appears for no apparent reason.

When melasma is related to pregnancy, the lesions usually gradually become lighter in the months following the pregnancy.

Melasma.

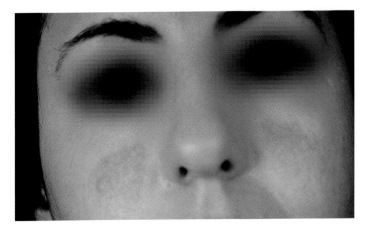

Note: Before using bleaching preparations for melasma there are two essential steps to be taken:

- minimizing exposure to the sun;
- because certain hormonal or other medications can cause or aggravate the melasma, a dermatologist should be consulted with regard to stopping certain medications.

Post-inflammatory pigmented lesions

Hyperpigmented areas of skin may appear following some types of skin inflammation, such as:

- acne
- contact dermatitis
- trauma or burns to the skin

In these cases, treatment with a bleaching agent is of limited value, since the pigment has 'sunk' into the deeper layers of the skin. The earlier treatment is started following the initial insult to the skin, the better the chances are for improvement.

Berloque dermatitis

A unique form of pigmentation of the skin is seen in the skin inflammation known as **Berloque dermatitis**. The pigmented area is irregular in shape; the common sites of occurrence are on the sides of the neck, behind the ears, and on the cheeks. The problem occurs as a result of the use of perfumes and aftershave lotion. These preparations contain substances called **furocoumarins**. The application of these compounds, combined with exposure to the sun, results in the pigmented areas of Berloque dermatitis. In this condition, skin lesions appear as dark-toned irregular blotches. These compounds do not cause any damage when the skin is not exposed to the sun.

General remarks regarding bleaching preparations

Most cosmetic problems leading to hyperpigmentation are related to sun exposure. Therefore, when using bleaching preparations, the sun should be avoided as much as possible. If it is impossible to totally prevent exposure to the sun, it is worthwhile using a sunscreen when outdoors (some bleaching preparations already incorporate a sunscreen).

Bleaching preparations are meant to be applied only to the hyperpigmented skin. There is obviously no point in bleaching the normal, light skin adjacent to the hyperpigmented area. If the distribution of the hyperpigmented blotches is such that it is impossible to apply the preparation without some of it getting onto the normal skin, a dermatologist should be consulted. The dermatologist may be able to suggest a more effective form of treatment, aimed only at the pigmented areas. For example, this may involve treatment such as freezing the lesion with liquid nitrogen.

It could take months before any improvement in the skin can be discerned. The efficacy of a bleaching preparation and its rapidity of action depend on the nature of the active ingredients it contains, and the type of lesion being treated.

More than one bleaching agent can be used for any given lesion. For example, hyperpigmented blotches may be treated with two different preparations – one to be used in the morning, and a different one for nighttime. The rationale of this approach is that different preparations exert their bleaching effect by different mechanisms. In addition, this approach provides a complementary treatment in cases where one of the preparations (such as retinoic acid) cannot be used during daylight. Furthermore, a mixture of preparations containing more than one active ingredient may be used. A common combination used by dermatologists, for example, is composed of **hydroquinone and retinoic acid**.

Note: All these treatments must be performed only under a physician's instructions

Bleaching preparations

Hydroquinone
Hydroquinone is a well-accepted agent for bleaching hyperpigmented lesions. It slows down and prevents the production of melanin in the skin.

The product is available in the USA in concentrations of up to 4%. In concentrations up to 2%, it can be purchased over the counter without a prescription. Products based on hydroquinone in concentrations of 4% can only be purchased with a doctor's prescription. At higher concentrations, above 5%, there is an increased risk of skin irritation (manifested by reddening and itching of the skin and a burning sensation) – without the higher concentration achieving any greater bleaching effect than the lower concentrations.

In the European Community hydroquinone is no longer permitted to be purchased over the counter; it is available by prescription only.

Mode of use
The preparation should be applied twice a day – in the morning and before retiring to bed. The hydroquinone may be combined with a sunscreen agent (this is recommended). The preparation may be based on hydroquinone alone, or may be a combination of hydroquinone with other bleaching agents or with corticosteroid compounds.

Efficacy
Following a minimum several weeks of treatment, one can usually discern some bleaching of the lesions. The use of hydroquinone-based preparations results in improvement in 70–80% of patients. In some cases, the use of

hydroquinone does not have any beneficial effect. Once the affected skin has faded to the desired shade, the preparation should be discontinued, but sunscreen should still be applied. Note that the bleaching effect may be only temporary, and after some time without treatment, the skin may darken again to its original shade. In this case, the following options should be considered by the physician:

- the use of a preparation with a higher concentration of hydroquinone;
- combination of hydroquinone with other bleaching agents (this is usually the preferred option).

Adverse effects

- Hydroquinone may tint the nails orange. Contact with the nails should be avoided while using hydroquinone.
- Not commonly, one may notice irritation of the skin following the use of hydroquinone, manifested by an itching sensation and redness. In such a case, the treatment should be discontinued and a physician consulted.

Hydroquinone monobenzyl ether (HMBE)

Hydroquinone monobenzyl ether is chemically similar to hydroquinone; but when applied to the skin, the effect cannot be controlled:

- the bleaching may occur in areas away from where it was applied;
- the bleaching continues for several months after the patient has stopped using the product.

Therefore this agent is not to be used for bleaching dark, hyperpigmented skin lesions.

The only use for HMBE is in the disease known as **vitiligo**, where the condition is widespread over large areas of skin. In vitiligo, hypopigmented white blotches appear on the skin for reasons that are not clear. In vitiligo, there is a defect in the function of the immunological system that interferes with the formation of skin pigment. Since the white blotches in vitiligo cannot be darkened, the only way to achieve a more or less uniform skin colour is to bleach unaffected (normal) areas of skin using HMBE. The entire skin becomes hypopigmented – however at least it is all the same colour. Obviously this treatment requires close medical supervision.

Retinoic acid

The effect of retinoic acid on ageing of the skin and on acne lesions has been described and explained in Chapters 8, 9 and 16. This substance, alone or combined with other products, has some effect on bleaching dark, hyperpigmented skin blotches. Preparations based on retinoic acid are available (by prescription only) in concentrations of 0.025%, 0.05% and 0.1%.

Azelaic acid

Azelaic acid inhibits the production of melanin in the skin; it can therefore be used for bleaching hyperpigmented skin lesions. Preparations containing azelaic acid are available in concentrations of 10%, 20% and 35%, and are applied twice daily for several months. Azelaic acid is reported to result in improvement in approximately 70% of patients within five months of starting treatment. This compound is also used by dermatologists for treating acne. It may only be prescribed by a physician.

How did the treatment arise?

The idea of using azelaic acid for bleaching hyperpigmented skin arose because of a known phenomenon seen in a fungal infection of the skin called **pityriasis vesicolor**. In this condition, pale blotches appear on the skin. These are attributed to the presence of azelaic acid in the affected areas. It therefore seemed logical to use azelaic acid to deliberately bleach hyperpigmented skin. In various research studies, the product was indeed found to be somewhat effective.

Alpha-hydroxy acids

Alpha-hydroxy acids have some effect on bleaching skin and bleaching hyperpigmented skin lesions. In the past, skin bleaching properties were attributed to extracts of certain fruits and vegetables (particularly cucumbers, lemons and strawberries). If indeed there is some bleaching of dark skin following the use of fruit and vegetable extracts, it may be due to the presence of alpha-hydroxy acids in these extracts. Alpha-hydroxy acids are dealt with in more detail in Chapter 17. (See the photograph on page 192.)

Other preparations used for bleaching hyperpigmented blotches

Other substances that are said to be able to bleach hyperpigmented skin are:

- *Glycerrhiza glabra*;
- liquorice extract – from the root of the liquorice plant;
- kojic acid – this substance is derived from yeast, and prevents the production of melanin in the skin (it was originally developed by the Japanese cosmetic industry, and subsequently appeared in other parts of the world).

Additional compounds for bleaching of dark skin blotches have recently emerged from the cosmetics industry; because these are relatively new, it is still difficult to assess their efficacy. It can be assumed that those found to be effective will in time join the preparations available today. Among these new compounds, we mention the following:

- arbutin
- 4-thioresorcin

various plant extracts, such as:

- *Catharanthus roseus*
- *Chamomilla recutita*
- ganoderma
- green tea (*Theaceae*)

Decades ago, the accepted treatment for bleaching skin lesions included products containing mercury salts. Their use is now prohibited because of their potential adverse effects – these substances are highly toxic. Hydrogen peroxide can also bleach melanin by oxidizing it, but it is not usually used for bleaching of skin since it may cause skin irritation. The main use of hydrogen peroxide is for bleaching hair.

Other forms of treatment that can be performed by a physician

Dermatologists may use other chemical and physical treatments. These treatments may, in many cases, be more effective than the treatments described hitherto, depending on the nature of the skin problem. Of the many treatments in use, we mention the following:

- freezing using liquid nitrogen
- laser treatment
- trichloroacetic acid (TCA)

The dermatologist decides which particular form of treatment to use for which lesion and hyperpigmented area, depending on the type of skin problem and the medical background of the patient. Take, for example, 'sun spots', as described earlier in the chapter. Because of the distribution of these small, isolated spots on the back of the hand, on a background of large areas of normal skin, the treatment of choice would seem to be to spray and freeze each lesion separately using liquid nitrogen (this is done by a dermatologist). This treatment is often preferable to the long-term application of skin-bleaching substances to the back of the hand, which, in fact, is mostly normal-coloured skin.

Note that skin-peeling treatments may also be effective in the treatment of dark blotches. The degree of improvement depends mainly on the depth of the peeling, the peeling preparation used, the type of skin lesion, and the extent of its pigmentation. Chemical peeling of skin is discussed in detail in Chapter 22.

Summary

Dark lesions of the skin are known in medical parlance as hyperpigmented lesions, and may include freckles, 'sun spots', the 'pregnancy mask' and other lesions.

Various substances are used in the treatment of hyperpigmented skin lesions: hydroquinone, retinoic acid, alpha-hydroxy acids, *Glycerrhiza glabra*, liquorice extract and kojic acid, among others. Each substance can be used separately, or can be combined with other substances – for example with one being used in the morning and another in the evening.

Whenever hyperpigmented lesions appear on the skin, the patient must:

- minimize exposure to the sun
- consult a dermatologist

19

Astringents

Contents   What are astringents, and what are they used for? •
Composition of astringents • Comments

What are astringents, and what are they used for?

Astringents are used to:

- give the skin a 'taut', cool, refreshing feeling
- temporarily constrict the skin pores
- remove the outer layer of oil from the skin

Astringents have many other names in the cosmetics industry. They are also
called, for example, 'skin tonics', or 'skin toners'. Astringents usually come as
solutions, although some are in the form of gels.

Astringents are applied following skin cleansing. The commonest form of
astringent, as a cosmetic, is in aftershave products.

Note: Not all the claims made about astringents have been tested scientifically. The question of how beneficial they really are for the skin is unan-
swered. We assume that their benefit to the skin varies depending on the
nature of the specific product, and the type of skin it is used on.

Composition of astringents

Astringents are solutions containing a mixture of **alcohol and water** in various
proportions. Astringents for use on dry skin should contain minimal concentrations of alcohol (which tends to dry out the skin). For very dry skin, an
astringent containing moisturizers should be used. On the other hand, astringents for use on oily skin have a higher concentration of alcohol.

Astringents usually contain **aluminium** or **zinc salts**, which are said to constrict the skin pores. This effect has not been tested scientifically. Should it be

correct, there may well be some advantage to constricting the skin pores following cleansing of the face, in order to prevent the entry of dirt, particles of soot and dust into the pores.

Astringent solutions generally contain substances that cool and refresh, such as **menthol** or **camphor**. These substances have some kind of a 'medical fragrance' about them. Alcohol also gives a feeling of coolness because of its rapid evaporation from the skin. The solutions may also contain **dyes** and **fragrances**.

Sometimes **'exotic ingredients'**, derived from plants, that give the skin a 'taut', fresh, cool feeling, may be included. Witch hazel extract, for example, is derived from the leaves of the *Hamamelis Virginiana* tree, found in North America. This extract has anti-inflammatory properties. Because of its reputed astringent properties, it is a common ingredient in astringents and aftershave preparations. Other plants whose extracts are said to have astringent effects include species of oak (*Quercus*), where an extract is produced from its bark; or *Tilia*, where the extract is derived from the flowers.

Comments

The use of astringents following cleansing of the face once had an additional purpose – they helped to remove soap remnants left on the skin. Nowadays, with the increasing use of modern soaps ('soapless' soaps), rinsing the face with water is usually sufficient to remove any residual soap completely, so that this function of the astringent is unnecessary.

Aftershave preparations are made up of the same substances as are astringents; they also contain water and alcohol. The assumption is that even the low concentration of alcohol present in an aftershave has some antiseptic effect, which is helpful in dealing with tiny cuts or abrasions in the skin (some of them not even visible or felt) that occur during shaving. Again here, zinc or aluminium salts are said to constrict the skin pores that were dilated following rinsing of the face with warm water. Aftershave lotions give a feeling of freshness and coolness – usually due to the addition of menthol.

With regard to aftershave preparations, the only real difference between the various brands is the unique scent of each one.

It should be noted that the real practical value of astringents is controversial. It has not yet been shown in the medical literature that they indeed have any beneficial effect.

20
Preparations used in dermatology

Contents Overview • Antibiotics • Antifungal agents • Antiseptics • Preparations containing corticosteroids

Note: This chapter provides information about commonly used preparations. It is not intended that anyone not authorized to do so should treat him/herself or anybody else on the basis of the information in this chapter. In any case of skin disease, a physician should be consulted.

Overview

In the average family medicine cabinet, one can usually find remnants of various substances widely used in dermatology. Too often, people try to 'treat' skin lesions with these preparations, without having the appropriate, relevant knowledge. Treatment with an incorrect preparation may make the skin problem worse. Sometimes, it may make it difficult for the physician to arrive at an appropriate diagnosis and treat the patient correctly. For example, using a corticosteroid-containing cream to treat a skin lesion that is caused by a fungus will 'mask' and alter the clinical appearance, so that even an experienced physician may not be able to diagnose the problem correctly. In this chapter, we limit our discussion to those agents that are the most widely used:

- preparations used for treating skin infections (both bacterial and fungal)
- preparations containing corticosteroids

These substances are familiar to most of us. From experience, they also happen to be the substances that statistically are misused the most; it is to be hoped that basic knowledge about them may reduce the incidence of their misuse.

Antibiotics

Antibiotics are active against bacteria. These medications can kill bacteria or inhibit their growth. Common to all antibiotics is the fact that they are produced from various bacteria or certain fungi (moulds); most of the other antibacterial agents, such as antiseptics, are produced synthetically.

Antibiotics work in various ways. Commonly, their activity is accomplished by damaging and breaking the cell wall of the bacteria, or by interfering with the production of certain essential substances that the bacteria require. Antibiotics may be taken by mouth (tablets, capsules, syrups), injected into a muscle, or they may be infused into a vein (an intravenous infusion).

Antibiotics for use on the skin are usually in the form of solutions, creams or ointments. They are used for skin lesions infected by bacteria. The following are some examples of antibiotic agents for application to the skin:

bacitracin	fusidic acid	neomycin
chloramphenicol	gentamicin	oxytetracycline
chlortetracycline	mupirocin	tetracycline

For antibiotics used in the treatment of acne, see Chapter 9.

Antifungal agents

The substances listed here are for the treatment of skin infections caused by fungi. The commonest mode of action of these antifungal agents (but not of all of them) is by interfering with the production of substances that the fungus needs to build its cell wall. As a result, the cell wall develops 'holes', which stop the growth of the fungus and eventually lead to its death. The substances are divided into several groups, depending on their chemical composition:

- substances made up of compounds from the **imidazole group:**
bifonazole	isoconazole
clotrimazole	ketoconazole
econazole	miconazole
- Substances in which the active ingredient is **ciclopiroxolamine:**
- Other agents:
nystatin	tolnaftate
terbinafine	zinc undecylenate

These antifungal agents may be applied in the form of a solution, a cream, a shampoo, a powder, or another form, depending on the region to be treated.

Note that there are combinations of substances that contain corticosteroids or antibiotics in addition to the antifungal agent. These are used in cases where:

- there is both a fungal and a bacterial infection;
- the fungal infection has caused severe inflammation of the skin, in which case the use of an agent containing a steroid is advisable.

It should be remembered that different skin diseases may produce a clinical picture suggestive of a fungal infection. Inappropriate use of an antifungal agent on a skin lesion that is not necessarily a fungal infection may aggravate the condition. In spite of the fact that some of the substances listed above can be purchased without a doctor's prescription, it is advisable to use them only on a physician's advice.

Antiseptics

General comments
Antiseptics are substances that kill or inhibit the growth of bacteria and other microorganisms.

Antibacterial agents can be divided into two groups:

- **Bacteriostatics** inhibit the growth of bacteria.
- **Bactericidals** kill bacteria directly.

Most of the substances referred to here are bacteriostatic at low concentrations and bactericidal at high concentrations.

Types of antiseptics

Antiseptics for handwashing and disinfecting the skin before medical treatment
These include:

- hexachlorophene
- chlorhexidine
- high-concentration alcohol solutions

High-concentration alcohol solutions have very effective antiseptic properties. Consequently, alcohol solutions are widely used in cosmetic clinics, medical clinics and hospitals. Alcohol in a concentration of 70% is used to disinfect the skin prior to medical procedures. In addition, medical instruments are disinfected by soaking in concentrated solutions of alcohol.

Note: Certain cleansing agents, in high concentrations, can kill bacteria effectively – for example, quaternary ammonium compounds, which belong to the cationic surfactant group. **Cetrimide**, which belongs to that group, in low concentrations is a component of hair shampoos, and in higher concentrations it is a potent antiseptic used mainly for disinfecting medical instruments.

Antiseptic agents for treating infected areas of skin

These antiseptics are used in the form of solutions, in which the active ingredient is present in low concentrations – for example, solutions of **potassium permanganate** or solutions based on **chlorine.**

Weak solutions of potassium permanganate are pink/purple in colour. They are used for infected areas of skin, particularly weeping skin. For example, for an infection on a limb, the limb can be soaked in a potassium permanganate solution for several minutes, two to three times a day. Another method of treating infected weeping skin is by wetting the area repeatedly; a cotton cloth soaked in the antiseptic solution is placed on the infected area for a few minutes, two or three times a day.

Diluted chlorine solutions can also be used for wetting the affected areas.

Hydrogen peroxide

Hydrogen peroxide is a strong antiseptic, which comes as dilute solutions in water. Because hydrogen peroxide itself can damage body tissues, it is not normally used as a disinfectant.

Hydrogen peroxide is also used to bleach hair.

Iodine-based solutions

It is not clear exactly how iodine kills bacteria and other microorganisms, but it is effective and rapid in its action. It is available in the following forms:

- **Iodoform** is a compound that releases iodine and has a relatively weak antibacterial effect.
- **Povidone iodine** is a mixture of iodine with a polymer that releases the iodine slowly. It is available as a powder, an ointment, or a lotion of yellow–brown colour. Povidone iodine compounds are used for the treatment of infected

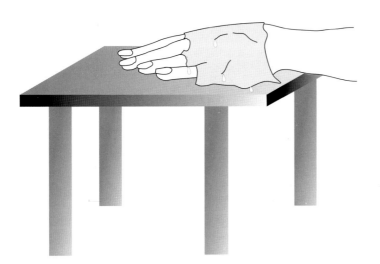

Wetting infected skin with a cotton cloth soaked in a solution of potassium permanganate.

areas of skin. In liquid form, they are also used as antiseptic preparations prior to medical procedures. Before use, it is advisable to determine whether the preparation about to be used contains alcohol. If it does, it should not be used on an open wound, since it may cause a severe burning sensation and, to a certain extent, may lead to tissue damage. Those povidone iodine compounds that contain alcohol are best reserved for use as antiseptic preparations prior to medical procedures.

- **Tincture of iodine** is based on iodine diluted with alcohol, and is used for the purposes mentioned above.

Synthetic dyes

These include **gentian violet** and **brilliant green**. These are synthetic dyes that were used for many years as antibacterial preparations. They have been replaced by the newer substances discussed above.

Preparations containing corticosteroids

Steroids (or **corticosteroids** or **glucocorticoids**) is the general name given to a group of hormones that are produced naturally in the body; some are produced in the adrenal gland, which is situated on top of the kidney. Among their many important functions is their anti-inflammatory activity, which is why they have been widely used in dermatological preparations for the treatment of inflammatory diseases of the skin.

Corticosteroids may be given by mouth, or injected into a muscle or a vein. In addition, corticosteroid preparations can be applied to an affected area of skin. As stated, dermatologists have available a wide range of preparations that contain corticosteroids of varying degrees of potency, which can be selected depending on the degree of skin inflammation. They can produce unwanted side-effects, particularly if used for long periods of time. Side-effects on the skin include the following:

- The skin may become thin and 'fragile' – the medical term is skin **atrophy**.
- **Purpura** – small areas of bleeding within the skin – can appear.
- Acne may appear as a result of prolonged corticosteroid usage – this is called **steroid acne**.
- **Telangiectases** – a network of fine blood vessels on the skin may appear (this is sometimes called 'couperose').
- There may be **hirsutism** – an increase in the amount of hair in the steroid-treated area.

Because of these potential side-effects, corticosteroids should not be used indiscriminately or without medical consultation. In many countries, including the USA and the UK, only preparations that contain a low concentration of hydrocortisone (0.5–1%) may be purchased over the counter – other corticosteroid preparations are available by prescription only. The duration of the

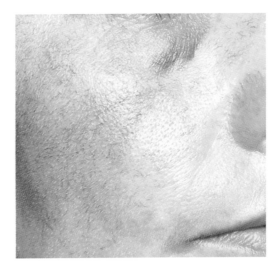

Purpura and telangiectasia following prolonged use of steroidal preparations.

Telangiectasia following prolonged use of steroidal preparations.

treatment must be determined by the physician, and steroids must never be used for longer than the recommended period. Furthermore,

- corticosteroid-containing preparations should not be **over-used** on the face, even with a relatively 'weak' steroid;
- a preparation containing a 'strong' corticosteroid may be absorbed through the skin into the blood, and as a result, not only may there be deleterious effects on the skin, but there may be generalized (systemic) effects on the body.

As stated earlier, there is a wide variety of corticosteroid preparations with different strengths. The main factor determining the strength is the type and concentration of steroid they contain. However, there are other factors involved, such as the nature of the preparation itself; thus, for example, an ointment is more potent than a cream containing the same corticosteroid.

In the following table, these preparations are divided into seven degrees of potency. Class I includes the 'very potent' preparations, while Class VII includes the 'weak' preparations. The use of any of these substances requires a dermatologist's advice. This is particularly important when dealing with the 'potent' corticosteroids – but even the 'weak' preparations should not be used for prolonged periods. This is especially important when they are applied to the face.

	Generic name	Examples of brand names
I	Clobetasol dipropionate 0.05%	Dermovate (ointment/cream)
	Clobetasol dipropionate 0.05%	Temovate (ointment/cream)
	Halobetasol dipropionate 0.05%	Ultravate (ointment)
	Betamethasone dipropionate 0.05%	Betnovate (cream)
	Betamethasone dipropionate 0.05%	Diprolene (ointment)
II	Clobetasole dipropionate 0.05%	Temovate scalp (solution)
	Betamethasone dipropionate 0.05%	Diprolene (cream)
	Betamethasone dipropionate 0.05%	Diprosone (ointment)
	Mometasone furoate %	Elocon (ointment)
	Fluocinonide 0.05%	Fluonex (cream)
	Halcinonide 0.1%	Halciderm Topical (cream)
	Halcinonide 0.1%	Halog (cream)
	Halcinonide 0.1%	Halog-E (ointment)
	Fluocinonide 0.05%	Lidex (cream)
	Betamethasone dipropionate 0.05%	Maxivate (ointment)
	Betamethasone dipropionate 0.05%	Psorion (ointment)
	Desoximetasone 0.25%	Topicort (cream)
III	Betamethasone dipropionate 0.05%	Aiphatrex (ointment)
	Triamcinolone acetonide 0.5%	Aristocort (ointment/cream)
	Amcininide 0.1%	Cyclocort (cream)
	Betamethasone dipropionate 0.05%	Diprosone (cream)
	Diflorasone diacetate 0.05%	Florone (cream)
	Diflorasone diacetate 0.05%	Florone E (ointment)
	Halcinonide 0.1%	Halog (cream)
	Triamcinolone acetonide 0.5%	Kenalog (cream)
	Fluocinonide 0.05%	Lidex E (cream)

Generic name	Examples of brand names
Difiorasone diacetate 0.05%	Maxiflor (cream)
Betamethasone dipropionate 0.05%	Maxivate (ointment)
Betamethasone dipropionate 0.05%	Psorcon (ointment)
IV Triamcinolone acetonide 0.1%	Adcortyl (cream)
Triamcinolone acetonide 0.1%	Aristocort (ointment/cream)
Triamcinolone acetonide 0.1%	Kenalog (cream)
Triamcinolone acetonide 0.1%	Kenalog H (ointment)
Triamcinolone acetonide 0.1%	Ledercort (cream)
Mometasone furoate 0.1%	Elocon (cream)
Halcinonide 0.025%	Halog (cream)
Fluocinolone acetonide 0.2%	Synalar HP (ointment)
Desoximetasone 0.05%	Topicort LP (cream)
V Betamethasone valerate 0.1%	Betatrex (ointment)
Ciocortolone pivalate 0.1%	Cloderm (ointment)
Fluticasone propionate 0.05%	Cutivate (ointment)
Hydrocortisone butyrate 0.1%	Locoid (ointment)
Fluocinolone acetonide 0.025%	Synalar (ointment)
Betametasone benzoate 0.025%	UtiCort (ointment)
Betamethasone valerate 0.1%	Valisone (ointment)
Hydrocortisone valerate 0.2%	Westcort (ointment)
VI Alclomethasone dipropionate 0.05%	Aclovate (ointment)
Triamcinolone acetonide 0.025%	Aristocort (ointment/cream)
Desonide 0.05%	DesOwen (ointment)
Triamcinolone acetonide 0.025%	Kenalog (cream)
Fluocinolone acetonide 0.01%	Synalar (cream)
Desonide 0.05%	Tridesilon (ointment)
Betamethasone valerate 0.01%	Valisone (ointment)
VII Hydrocortisone 1%	Acticort-100 (lotion)
Hydrocortisone 1% + urea 10%	Alphaderm (ointment)
Hydrocortisone 1%	Anusol HC (ointment)
Hydrocortisone 1%	Bactine HC (ointment)
Hydrocortisone 0.5%	Caldecort (ointment/cream)
Hydrocortisone 1% + urea 10%	Alphaderm (cream)
Hydrocortisone 1% + urea 10%	Calmurid HC (cream)
Hydrocortisone 1% + urea 10%	Carmol HC
Hydrocortisone 0.25%, 0.5%, 1%	Cetacort (lotion)

Generic name	Examples of brand names
Hydrocortisone 0.5%	Cortaid (ointment/cream/lotion)
Hydrocortisone 0.25%, 0.5%, 1%	CortoDome (ointment/lotion)
Hydrocortisone 1%	Dermacort (ointment/lotion)
Hydrocortisone 1%	Dermol HC (ointment/cream)
Hydrocortisone 1%, 2.5%	Eldecort (ointment/cream)
Hydrocortisone 1%, 2.5%	Hytone (cream/ointment/lotion)
Hydrocortisone 0.5%, 1%, 2.5%	Lacticare HC (lotion)
Hydrocortisone 0.5%	Lanacort (cream)
Hydrocortisone 1%	Nutracort (ointment/lotion)
Hydrocortisone 1%	PeneCort (solution)
Hydrocortisone 1%, 2.5%	SyneCort (ointment)
Hydrocortisone 1%	TexaCort (solution)

This table is reproduced by courtesy of Dr Alex Zvulunov.

21
Liposomes

Contents General background: are liposomes necessary? • The structure of cell membranes; phospholipids • What are liposomes? • The basis for the use of liposomes • What substances do liposomes contain? • Are liposomes effective? • Additional possible benefits of liposomes • Conclusion

General background: are liposomes necessary?

The term **liposome** has become more and more popular in the area of cosmetics. In many cases, a salesgirl at a cosmetics counter will advise her customers to purchase a certain product claiming that 'it contains liposomes'.

To understand what liposomes are, we must clarify some basic concepts about how substances penetrate the skin. The main barrier to the passage of substances from the exterior into the epidermis is the keratinous (horny) layer. These outer cells are arranged in compact layers, and contain large amounts of horny matter. Liposomes are used in an attempt to create a new method for transferring active products into the epidermis and dermis.

Penetration of substances into the skin

The major factor that determines the penetrating ability of substances into the skin is the **molecule size**. Beyond a certain size, molecules cannot penetrate the skin – only relatively small molecules can do so. For example, collagen, which is present in many cosmetic products, has relatively large molecules that cannot penetrate the skin.

In addition, oily products tend to penetrate the skin more easily than water-based preparations. Substances with better oil-solubility can penetrate better into the skin.

The structure of cell membranes; phospholipids

The external membranes of the cells, including skin cells, are made up of phospholipids, polysaccharides and various proteins. **Phospholipids** are fatty

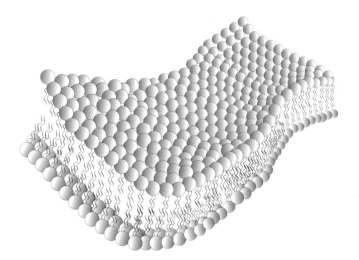

The cell membrane is formed of two layers of phospholipids.

compounds that contain phosphorus, and form the cell membrane as a two-layered structure. This structural organization prevents the passage of unwanted substances into, or out of, the cell, and allows the cell to regulate the entry and exit of various substances.

What are liposomes?

Liposomes are spherical vesicles, with a water-filled centre. Their diameter is measured in micrometres (microns, i.e. several thousandths of a millimetre). The membranes that form the spherical structure are composed of one or numerous layers.

A three-dimensional, monolayer liposome.

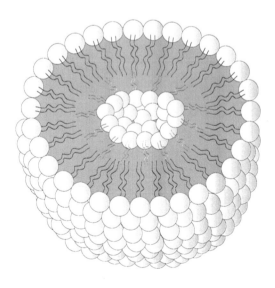

Multilamellar   Unilamellar

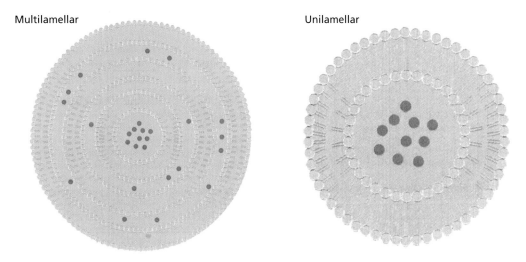

Various medications (marked in red) can be inserted into liposome vesicles. Liposomes can be **unilamellar** *(composed of one layer), or* **multilamellar** *(many-layered).*

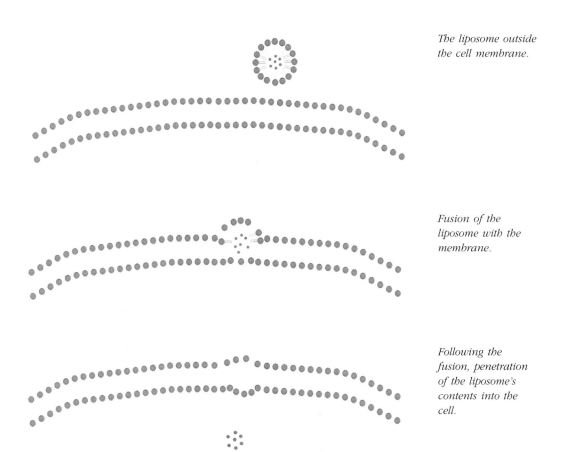

The liposome outside the cell membrane.

Fusion of the liposome with the membrane.

Following the fusion, penetration of the liposome's contents into the cell.

The basis for the use of liposomes

The basic idea derives from the fact that the cell membranes of the body (and the skin, of course) are composed of phospholipids. Therefore a small spherical liposome, itself composed of phospholipids, can serve as a carrier for active substances. Substances, such as medications, can be inserted into liposomes. An active product can be inserted to the liposome's core, or it can be anchored to the membrane surface.

In practical terms, it is not yet clear how this transport is achieved. One possible mechanism of transport and delivery would be fusing of the liposome membrane with the cell membrane, thereby allowing penetration into a skin cell. It is not clear whether this hypothetical mechanism is true. Most studies show that liposomes are destroyed on the skin surface, or in the outer horny layer. From here active substances can progress deeper into the skin – each substance penetrating according to its individual properties. Other studies raise the possibility that, because of the difficulty encountered in penetrating the horny layer, most of the liposomes enter the skin through skin pores.

What substances do liposomes contain?

In dermatology, antifungal medications are the main area of use for liposomes. Liposomes are currently also being investigated with regard to their use with antibiotics, corticosteroids and retinoids.

The major focus concerning liposomes is currently the cosmetics industry, because of the marketing allure they possess. Whether this allure is justified has yet to be established. The debate may soon be resolved, since many studies are currently researching liposomes and their advantages.

One can reasonably assume that collagen and elastin molecules are too large to penetrate the skin, and their insertion into liposomes is not likely to cause them to shrink. However, substances with smaller molecules may penetrate the skin more efficiently.

The cosmetics industry utilizes liposomes mostly for moisturizers. In addition, products containing various vitamins have been created. However, the value of these, whether or not they are enveloped in liposomes, is controversial.

New systems: niosomes

In order to increase the ability to penetrate the skin, niosomes were developed. The full scientific term is **non-ionic surfactant vesicles**. They are similar in composition to liposomes, and are spherically structured as well. The vesicle membranes of niosomes are composed of oily compounds of ether or alcohol.

Are liposomes effective?

Several studies have examined the efficacy of the liposomal system. An active product enveloped in liposomes was compared with the same product in a regular oil base. Some of the studies proved increased efficacy for the use of liposomes, especially regarding the oral use of certain medications. With regards to the topical use of drugs (i.e. drugs that are to be applied externally to the skin), the issue remains controversial.

Some scientists consider the issue a marketing gimmick for the cosmetic industry. Others perceive it as a significant turning point in cosmetics and dermatology. The issue is currently under investigation, so a definite conclusion concerning the efficacy of liposomes cannot yet be established.

Note that the main function of liposomes is to carry active ingredients into the skin. Therefore the potential beneficial effect of a preparation that contains liposomes is determined mainly by the biological properties of the specific ingredients that are carried by the liposomes.

Additional possible benefits of liposomes

Liposomes, composed of an oily substance, form a thin, oily film on the skin surface. There is a weak occlusive effect, and an increase in skin moisture. However, there is no significant advantage when compared with other moisturizers.

Contact between skin cells and active substances or topical medications decreases when these are enveloped in liposomes. This may decrease or modify allergic reactions.

Conclusion

Liposomes are not active substances in themselves. They act as a medium for penetration of active products in the skin. Their efficacy has yet to be established.

22

Chemical skin peeling

Contents Overview • For which problems is chemical skin peeling used?
• Skin depth and degrees of chemical peeling • Substances used in
chemical skin peeling • The depth of chemical skin peeling • Procedure
for chemical skin peeling • Level of pain with chemical skin peeling
• Course following chemical skin peeling • Possible complications of
chemical skin peeling and their management • Summary

Overview

Chemical skin peeling is a method of peeling the outer layers of the skin by
creating a chemical burn. As the burn heals, a new outer layer of skin forms.
The new skin that appears is smoother, pinker, tauter, and has a more uniform texture. After chemical peeling, 'sun spots' on the skin become paler.
Similarly, wrinkles are smoothed out to a certain extent, and some even disappear completely.

   We include a description of the technique of chemical peeling of the skin for
information and interest only. Under no circumstances do we suggest that
this technique be used for self-treatment. Skin peeling must only be performed by a physician experienced in the technique.

For which problems is chemical skin peeling used?

Chemical skin peeling is mainly used to treat solar damage in the form of 'sun
spots' (solar lentigines), and to smooth out the skin and eliminate wrinkles.
For fine wrinkles, superficial peeling is sufficient. For deeper wrinkles, such as
those found around the mouth and at the corners of the eyes, deeper peeling is
needed.

   Similarly, skin peeling can improve:

* other abnormalities of pigmentation, in the form of dark blotches on the
  face, such as the 'pregnancy mask' (melasma);
* superficial acne scars.

   Skin peeling is used for the above problems: it does not solve the problem of
thin skin that gives the face a 'droopy' look. In those cases, consideration

should be given to surgical treatment – a 'face lift' – which is performed by a plastic surgeon.

Skin depth and degrees of chemical peeling

- **Very superficial peeling** involves only the epidermis. There may be minimal involvement of the dermis.
- **Superficial peeling** includes the epidermis and the outermost part of the dermis.
- **Medium peeling** reaches the dermis, deeper than superficial peeling.
- **Deep peeling** reaches deeper into the dermis, to approximately half its depth.

The deeper the peeling reaches, the more significant is the influence on the facial skin. The possibility of lightening various blotches on the face increases substantially the deeper the peeling. With deeper peeling it is possible to erase wrinkles that are relatively deep and could not be treated with superficial peeling. Not infrequently, the procedure of superficial peeling has to be repeated several times until satisfactory results are obtained.

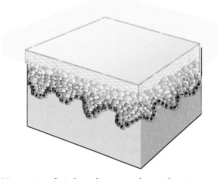

Very superficial peeling – only epidermis.

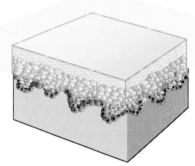

Superficial peeling – epidermis and outer dermis.

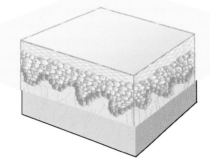

Medium peeling – deeper into the dermis.

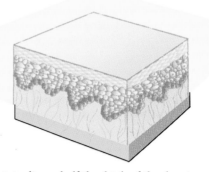

Deep peeling – half the depth of the dermis.

Regeneration of the skin following chemical peeling

If the peeling is superficial, the skin will regenerate from cells in the epidermis that replicate, multiply, and produce a new layer of epidermis.

How does the skin regenerate following deeper peeling, which reaches the dermis, since the epidermis is almost entirely destroyed? In these cases, the regeneration is mainly from cells coating the hair follicles, which go down quite deep into the dermis. Although these cells are situated 'deep' in the dermis, they are, in fact, epidermal cells. These cells replicate and divide until they cover the entire area that was denuded by the peeling. Within the dermis new collagen tissue forms, which replaces the collagen destroyed by the chemical treatment.

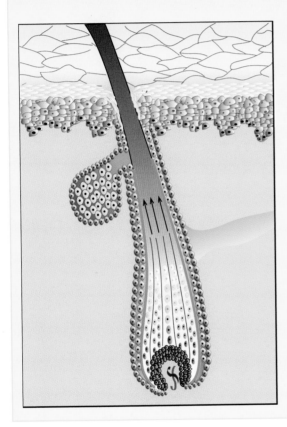

As this illustration shows, even at the depth of the dermis where the hair follicles extend, there are epidermal cells. It is from those cells that new skin regenerates following deep peeling.

Substances used in chemical skin peeling

The following are the substances most commonly used for chemical skin peeling:

- 'dry ice' (carbon dioxide snow)
- Jessner's solution, which contains resorcinol, salicylic acid and lactic acid

- alpha-hydroxy acids (see Chapter 17)
- trichloroacetic acid (TCA)
- phenol

As well as these, there are other substances that are used for chemical peeling; moreover, several substances can be mixed in a 'combination' product for peeling. Each physician selects an appropriate substance, depending on the depth of peeling to be achieved, the patient's skin type, and the physician's personal experience with that particular product.

The depth of chemical skin peeling

The major factors that determine the depth of the burn that results from peeling are:

- the chemical (or mixture of chemicals) used
- its concentration
- the length of time of contact with the skin
- whether an occlusive dressing is used

Apart from the above there are several other factors, such as:

- skin thickness
- the use of other preliminary treatments before peeling (such as the daily application of retinoic acid for about two weeks prior to chemical peeling)

Examples of preparations used for chemical skin peeling

Very superficial peeling may be performed using: 10–20% trichloroacetic acid, Jessner's solution or alpha-hydroxy acids (see Chapter 17).
Superficial peeling may be carried out using: 35% trichloroacetic acid or 50–70% alpha-hydroxy acids (see Chapter 17).
Medium peeling may be carried out using: 35% trichloroacetic acid combined with dry ice, or with Jessner's solution.
Deep peeling is usually carried out using phenol.
   There are many methods of skin peeling apart from those mentioned above. Each doctor uses the technique with which he/she feels most comfortable and with which he/she has had the most experience.

Procedure for chemical skin peeling

We shall describe the technique using trichloroacetic acid.

1 Cleansing

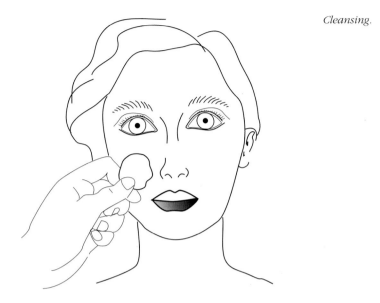

Cleansing.

2 Applying trichloroacetic acid to the skin using a cotton swab applicator

Within a short time, the skin develops a white–grey colour, because of the chemical destruction of the outer layers of the skin, as shown in the illustration.

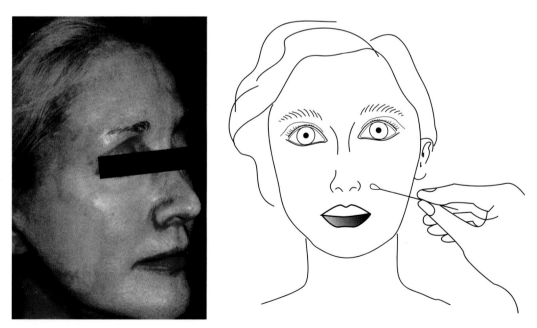

Applying trichloroacetic acid to the skin: following exposure to the trichloroacetic acid, the epidermis changes colour.

3 Rinsing the substance off after two minutes of skin contact
The patient will feel a certain degree of discomfort, depending on the concentration of the substance.

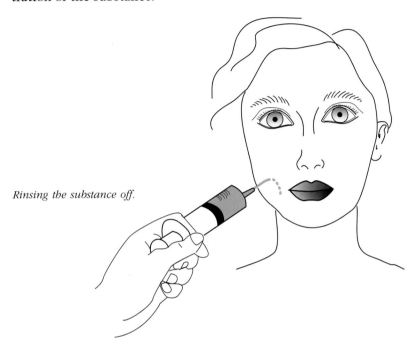

Rinsing the substance off.

Application of an occlusive dressing
Antibiotic cream may also be applied.

Preparation prior to chemical skin peeling

Many physicians recommend applying retinoic acid to the face at night for approximately two weeks prior to the skin peeling treatment. This preparatory treatment apparently improves the penetration of the active peeling substance into the skin, and the subsequent healing of the peeled area is quicker and more effective.

Dark-skinned patients should undergo preparation with skin bleaching agents prior to skin peeling. This prevents the appearance of dark pigmented areas of skin following the peeling treatment. One preparation commonly used for this purpose is **Kligman's solution**, which contains hydroquinone, hydrocortisone and retinoic acid. It must be applied daily for three weeks prior to skin peeling.

A month or so prior to the peeling, a 'spot test' should be performed using a small amount of the preparation to be used for the peeling. This test is carried out on area of skin that is not readily seen, such as behind the ear. Over the next few weeks, any untoward reaction to the substance (such as inflammation or darkening of the skin) will become obvious, in which case the chemical peeling treatment should not be carried out.

Level of pain with chemical skin peeling

Superficial skin peeling is associated with a mild burning sensation at the time of the treatment, which in most cases amounts to no more than mild discomfort.

Medium skin peeling (particularly if carried out with trichloroacetic acid) is associated with bearable pain during the treatment, which subsides quickly thereafter.

Deep peeling, using phenol, causes very severe pain during the treatment and for up to two days afterwards. The patient must be given intravenous analgesic medications, or general anaesthesia – depending on the physician's and patient's choice.

Course following chemical skin peeling

Superficial peeling

Superficial peeling, if performed only once, has almost no discernible effect, but if the treatment is repeated several times over a period of months, good results can be achieved. Shortly after the treatment, the skin becomes red, and within two days it develops a brown colouration. The mild burning sensation, which is transient, can be alleviated by applying cold compresses, or by directing a flow of cold air from a fan onto the skin. Within three to five days, the superficial layers of the skin start to peel. Healing is almost complete a week after the treatment. Overall, this treatment is simple, the risks are minimal, and healing is quick.

Superficial skin peeling can be repeated at short intervals (every few weeks) in order to achieve a deeper and deeper peel with each treatment.

Medium peeling

Redness of the skin appears approximately an hour after the treatment, and apart from cold compresses or a flow of cool air over the area, usually no further treatment is needed. Later, the face becomes swollen, and five to seven days later, the skin starts to peel. It takes about two weeks for healing to occur, at which time new, smooth, delicate skin covers the area. 'Sun spots' are much less obvious, and fine wrinkles become flattened out. The redness of the face lasts for a few weeks, and then gradually disappears.

Deep peeling

Healing following deep peeling is slower than that following superficial or medium peeling. The face becomes more swollen than following medium peeling, and the redness is much more obvious. The swelling and redness last for three to six months. During that period, the patient is unable to tolerate any cosmetics on the face, and they should not be used. Even dyeing the hair can cause severe itching.

Deep peeling can help in the elimination of relatively deep wrinkles around the mouth and eyes.

When should a physician avoid chemical skin peeling?

There are a number of situations in which a discerning physician will choose not to perform chemical skin peeling. Anyone falling into one of the following categories should not have this treatment:
- patients with a tendency to form excessive scarring;
- patients with relatively dark skin should only undertake superficial peeling;
- patients who are going to be exposed to the sun following the treatment (because of their occupation or because they are unlikely to follow instructions to avoid exposure);
- smokers should probably not undergo chemical skin peeling, since their skin healing is generally not as good as in non-smokers, they have a higher risk of skin infection following treatment, and wrinkles are more likely to recur;
- patients who are emotionally unstable or have exaggerated, unrealistic expectations of the outcome of treatments.

Possible complications of chemical skin peeling and their management

The complications of skin peeling are usually preventable and treatable, and an experienced physician knows how to avoid them. The more common complications include the following:

Bacterial infection
The risk of bacterial infection can be minimized by paying careful attention to correct treatment technique and by the patient following the physician's advice after the treatment. The more superficial the peeling, the less is the likelihood of infection.

Alterations in skin pigmentation
Skin colour which may become either paler or darker. Using concentrations of phenol that are too high can cause pale areas of skin to appear (hypopigmentation). Trichloroacetic acid, on the other hand, usually causes dark areas of pigmentation (hyperpigmentation). To minimize this risk:

- The physician should take care to use the appropriate concentrations of the peeling substance.
- The patient should be advised to avoid exposure to the sun after peeling.
- In patients with dark skin (who tend to develop hyperpigmentation following peeling), it is advisable to prepare the skin before treatment with skin bleaching agents.

Scarring
The commonest reason for the appearance of scars after peeling is infection (viral or bacterial) of skin that was not treated correctly. Meticulous care in

taking the appropriate preventive measures, and immediate and effective treatment at the first sign of infection, will significantly decrease the risk of scarring. Less commonly, scars can appear if the concentration of the peeling substance was inadvertently too high. A wise physician will prefer to use a concentration a little less than what is 'officially' recommended, in order to provide a safety margin to allow for possible errors in the preparation of the product. For example, using 60% phenol instead of 50% may have drastic effects on the skin.

Herpes virus infection in the peeled area

It is common practice to prevent this complication by routinely giving the patient antiviral medication orally, starting from the day prior to the treatment, until a few days after the treatment. The currently accepted treatment is with tablets containing **acyclovir**. Newer preparations for the prevention and treatment of viral infections include **famciclovir** and **valciclovir**.

Sensitivity to cold

Marked cold sensitivity of the face can occur following chemical peeling.

Prolonged redness, an itchy feeling, and intolerance to cosmetics

These may occur following chemical peeling.

Heart and kidney problems

There have been reports of complications involving disturbances of heart rhythm and possible kidney damage following the use of phenol for deep chemical peeling, because of absorption of the substance into the bloodstream. Therefore patients undergoing this treatment may need to be connected to a heart monitor to watch for possible alterations in the heart rhythm. They should also be given intravenous fluids to prevent kidney damage.

Effects of sunlight

Exposure to sunlight following a peeling procedure can cause changes in skin pigmentation, resulting in the appearance of dark blotches in the new skin that grows back following the peeling. Therefore the patient should be told to strictly avoid any exposure to sunlight following the treatment. The length of this period of strict avoidance of sunlight will vary, depending on the depth of peeling, and is determined by the physician. However, even after this period of strict, *total* avoidance of sunlight, it is still advisable to avoid sun exposure as much as possible. If it is impossible to totally avoid exposure to the sun, a high-level protective sunscreen should be used when outdoors.The skin that regrows following peeling is particularly delicate and sensitive, and the harmful effects of the sun's rays on skin are well known.

Avoidance of cosmetics

As stated previously, following deep peeling there is intolerance to cosmetic preparations, and the patient should be advised to refrain from applying cosmetics to the face for several weeks or months following chemical peeling, depending on the depth of the peeling.

Note: In older women who have solar damage to the skin, peeling treatment that is too effective may not be beneficial. The contrast between smooth facial skin, free of wrinkles, and the deeply wrinkled untreated skin of the neck, with sun spots scattered over it, is not an aesthetically desirable result.

Summary

Chemical skin peeling is a technique whereby the outer layers of the skin are peeled away by means of a chemical burn. The substances used to achieve chemical peeling include dry ice, Jessner's solution, alpha-hydroxy acids, trichloroacetic acid, phenol and other substances. Chemical skin peeling is used mainly to lighten dark skin blotches (such as 'sun spots'), and to smooth or eradicate wrinkles.

23

Laser treatment in dermatology: Cosmetic applications

Contents Overview: laser treatment of various lesions • Skin peeling using a laser • Hair removal using a laser • Summary

Overview: laser treatment of various lesions

The ability of laser instruments to treat a range of dermatological conditions is based on two basic properties of lasers:

- the ability of a laser to produce a powerful, focused light beam that precisely destroys the tissue being treated;
- the ability of a laser beam to 'home in' on a specific target, depending on the colour and other characteristics of the target tissue – this 'colour-specific' targeting ability significantly reduces damage to surrounding tissues whose colour differs from the target tissue.

It follows from the above that there are various types of laser instruments, designed to treat skin lesions of various colours; for example:

- a **ruby laser** may be effective in the treatment of certain skin lesions that have a blue or brown colouration;
- a **pulsed-dye laser** can be used to treat lesions that are very vascular (i.e. contain many blood vessels), and is therefore the appropriate instrument for treating fine networks of blood vessels (telangiectases) that appear on the skin, or various growths derived from blood vessels in the skin.

Apart from the above, there are lasers designed to treat a wide range of skin lesions, including warts caused by viruses, scars, and other skin tumours of various types.

Other uses of lasers, such as in facial skin peeling and hair removal, will be discussed in detail below.

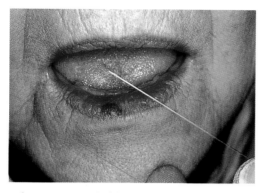
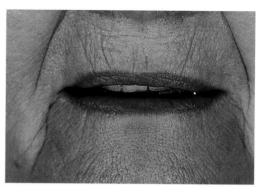

A lesion composed of blood vessels (the medical term is 'venous lake') before (left) and after (right) treatment with a laser.

Removing tattoos by laser

Tattoos result from dyes penetrating the skin. Lasers can selectively affect the dye material in the skin by 'bursting' the material into tiny particles, which are then engulfed by a special subgroup of white blood cells (called macrophages) in the tissues without causing any damage to the normal skin in the region. It is obvious that the laser used may be selected according to the colour(s) of the tattoo.

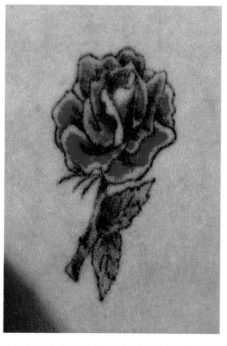
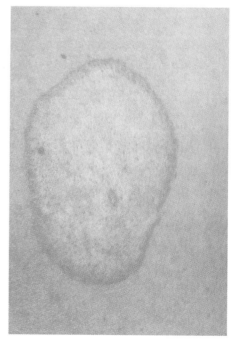

A tattoo, before (left) and after (right) laser treatment.

Skin peeling using a laser

The principle behind skin peeling using a laser is the same as that of chemical skin peeling. In both cases, the aim is to create a superficial burn on the skin of the face, so that as the burn wound heals, new 'rejuvenated' skin appears.

Until recently, lasers could not be used for skin peeling, because of the risk of causing a burn deeper than intended, since the depth of the burn could not be accurately controlled. However, advances in laser technology have led to the developments of laser instrumentation that can produce extremely short pulses (less than a thousandth of a second). This means that the actual time the beam is in contact with the skin is shorter, thus allowing lasers to be introduced for skin peeling. As a result of these technical advances the operator can now determine the precise depth in the skin to which the laser beam penetrates, and can therefore achieve exactly the depth of peeling required. The laser instruments used for this purpose are:

- the CO_2 laser
- the erbium : YAG (yttrium aluminium garnet) laser

The lasers mentioned above are mainly used for removing acne scars, and for the treatment of wrinkles around the eyes and mouth. Deeper wrinkles, resulting from movements of the facial muscles (such as wrinkles on the forehead or between the eyebrows) respond less well.

The beneficial effects of laser skin peeling last for a variable time, which differs from person to person. The possible side-effects of laser skin peeling are similar to those following chemical skin peeling. The main potential problems are redness of the face that may last up to three months following treatment, the development of scars and changes in the pigmentation (colour) of the skin.

Laser skin peeling is a safe procedure, provided that the operator is skilled and that the treatment is performed in line with accepted medical guidelines.

Hair removal using a laser

The idea of removing hair so that the treatment will be effective for long periods using laser technology was published in 1995. The scientific basis for this treatment is the fact that there is a difference in colour between the hair follicle and the skin; the light energy is directed towards the hair follicle. Since the laser beam 'homes in' on the dark pigment in the hair, the lighter the skin and the darker the hair, the more selectively will the laser affect the follicle and not the surrounding tissue. The laser beam damages the hair follicle so that no more hair can grow.

The main side-effects of this treatment are:

- a mild feeling of discomfort during treatment (this discomfort is bearable and does not require local anaesthetic);
- local redness, which may last from a few minutes to a few hours;
- superficial burns, usually resolving without leaving any residual sign.

The following important points should be noted:

- In view of the above, this treatment should not be used in people with dark skin. Light hairs cannot be treated by laser techniques. In the above cases, there is insufficient difference between the colour of the hair and the colour of the skin, which is what the laser treatment requires for it to be effective and safe. In dark-skinned people laser treatment may cause **hypopigmentation** – lightening of the skin around the hair follicle. In most cases, however, this phenomenon resolves by itself in time.
- Laser treatment arrests the active growth period of the treated hairs for long periods – sometimes for several years. The response varies according to the region of the body being treated: the results in the armpits, groin and legs are satisfactory; facial hairs are less responsive to laser treatment. The response to the treatment may also vary considerably from person to person, for reasons that are not fully understood. Some ten percent of the hairs require brief 'reinforcement' treatment two or three times a year.

The efficiency of laser treatment depends on which phase the treated hair is in

Lasers are effective for dealing with hair follicles that are in the growth phase (**anagen phase**). However, in the **telogen phase**, the hair that is about to degenerate is situated some distance from the place in the follicle from where the new hair will grow, so there is no point in cauterizing the telogen hair with a laser beam. (The phases of the life cycle of a hair are described in Chapter 25 on the structure of hair.)

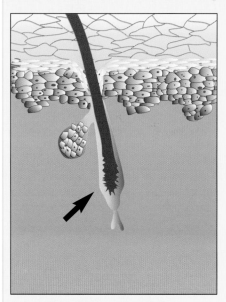

Telogen hair, about to degenerate

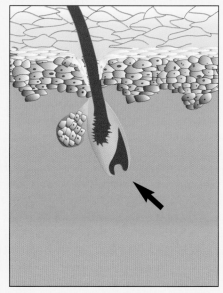

Next stage; the new hair begins to grow from another point (not treated by laser)

The results obtained to date from many patients are encouraging, and justify the continuing use of lasers for hair removal. It should be remembered that this technique is still in its infancy, and further developments and improvements can be expected.

Note that there are other devices on the market that have a similar mechanism of action to lasers: a beam of (non-laser) light is directed at and damages the hair follicle.

Summary

In spite of all the advantages of laser treatment discussed here, it should be remembered that the laser is not the definitive answer to all skin problems. Medical problems that require laser treatment must be distinguished from those that are best managed by other methods. For example:

- The recommended and accepted treatment for 'solar keratoses' is with 5-fluorouracil (5-FU) preparations or with liquid nitrogen, and not necessarily laser rays.
- A lesion that may be malignant must not be treated by a laser. In such cases, the lesion should be totally excised, together with a safety margin around it, and sent for microscopic examination. Moles (melanocytic naevi) should definitely not be treated by laser.
- In some cases, a doctor will prefer to perform skin peeling (for removing wrinkles in the skin) using a chemical peeling substance rather than a laser.

The laser should not be thought of as the be-all and end-all for cosmetic treatments.

24

Camouflaging skin lesions and other disfiguring conditions

Contents Overview • Types of skin lesions that can be hidden using makeup • Two techniques of camoufllage: foundation creams and cover creams • Foundation creams • Applying foundation cream • What are cover creams? • Matching cover creams to the skin • Applying cover cream • Determining the right application method for the three distinct types of skin • Recreating skin imperfections

Overview

This chapter deals with various ways of camouflaging skin lesions. The following pages describe a series of aesthetic problems that cannot always be treated effectively medically. The correct and efficient use of makeup techniques can help the patient considerably, and bring about a marked improvement in his/her appearance.

By reading this chapter, the reader will by no means be qualified to practise as an expert in makeup – that requires skills that take years of experience to acquire. Nevertheless, reading this chapter will provide some idea of the types of techniques in use, and the various possibilities that exist in the field of camouflaging skin lesions.

Before trying to 'hide' a skin lesion, it is recommended that a physician should be consulted:

- It is important to confirm the nature of the lesion to make sure it is not something that requires medical treatment. For example, the removal of cancerous lesions is of critical importance, and should be performed not just because of aesthetic considerations. Moreover, sometimes a skin lesion may be the sign of an internal disease. Merely covering up or hiding the lesion, without consulting a doctor, may delay appropriate diagnosis and treatment of the underlying illness.
- It must be determined whether there is some way of removing the lesion permanently (e.g. surgery, laser treatment, bleaching preparation, or some other technique), rather than merely hiding it.

Types of skin lesions that can be hidden using makeup

Pink–red lesions

Fine network of blood vessels
The medical term for a fine network of blood vessels is **telangiectasia**. (see Chapter 11). It is a relatively common condition, which is usually the result of cumulative damage to the skin from various causes: cumulative exposure to the sun, radiation therapy for various diseases, prolonged use of steroid-containing medications, and others. Sometimes these lesions are a manifestation of certain skin diseases.

Various growths derived from blood vessels
There is wide range of growths that are derived from the tissues that form blood vessels. Because these lesions contain a relatively large amount of blood they usually range from pink to red in colour. The term **angioma** is used to describe a group of benign growths that are derived from the tissues that make up the blood vessels. Although these growths are benign, and pose no medical danger to the patient, they may be very bothersome aesthetically.

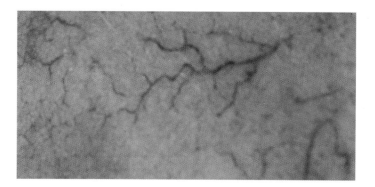

Telangiectasia of the face.

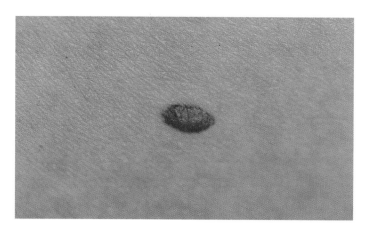

Angioma.

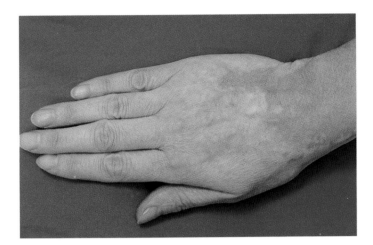

Vitiligo on the skin of the hands.

Light-coloured (hypopigmented) lesions

Vitiligo is a skin disease that is characterized by light, white/ivory-coloured lesions. The reason for the appearance of these areas on the skin is not really known, although we do know that in this disease there is some abnormality in the function of the body's immune system. As a result, the patient's immune system attacks his/her own pigment-producing system in the skin.

Another group of light-coloured skin lesions includes pale areas of skin that can appear following some inflammatory process or injury. The medical term for these areas is **post-inflammatory hypopigmentation**. Following injury or inflammation in a certain region, that area of skin may become paler (hypopigmented) – or sometimes darker (hyperpigmented).

Pale brown to dark lesions

A typical example of this type of lesion is the **'pregnancy mask'** (**melasma**, or **chloasma** in medical parlance). Melasma describes a specific distribution of brown pigmentation on the face, which is not infrequently seen in pregnant women. These are light to dark brown in colour. They are usually symmetrical in appearance, and occur typically on the upper lip, the forehead and the chin.

For a more detailed discussion of the 'pregnancy mask', see Chapter 18 on bleaching preparations.

Other pigmented lesions of the skin include **freckles**, **'sun spots'** ('liver spots', correctly termed **solar lentigenes**) and **naevi** ('beauty spots'). These lesions are discussed in more detail in Chapter 18 on bleaching preparations, and Chapter 14 on skin tumours.

Scars

Scars may range in colour from pale to dark. They may be raised above the skin surface, or sunken below the surface, so that when using makeup to 'hide' scars, these parameters must also be kept in mind.

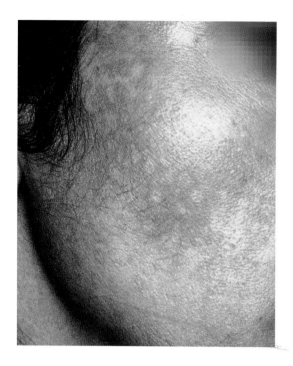

'Pregnancy mask' (melasma).

Transient problems

All the aesthetic problems mentioned above refer to lesions that are present on the skin for a long time. However, there may be transient injuries or lesions on the skin that are also an aesthetic problem and need to be dealt with by makeup and camouflage. For example, a blow or injury may produce a red, swollen area on the face. Concealing such a lesion would be desirable before some important social event, for instance.

In these cases also, it is important to consult a dermatologist before embarking on cosmetic treatment. In certain skin diseases, one should avoid applying makeup preparations on the affected skin areas.

Two techniques of camouflage: foundation creams and cover creams

Attracting attention away from facial or bodily disfigurements by camouflaging can be achieved by two different techniques. For cosmetic problems that require full concealment, one should use **cover creams**. On the other hand, a variety of skin lesions may require only subtle textural and pigment blending using **foundation creams**.

Selection of the cosmetic solution will depend on the quality of the cosmetic result that can be achieved by each technique, what the individual can and will apply, the cost of the materials, and how well the procedure fits into his/her daily activities.

It is advisable when deciding on the appropriate technique for camouflaging skin lesions to seek the advice of an experienced cosmetician or makeup expert.

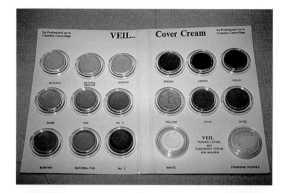

Two examples of cover cream palettes.

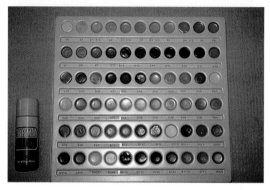

Foundation creams

There are two types of foundation creams:

- clear foundation cream that is applied in order to 'bind' makeup preparations to the skin;
- foundation creams that contain various colouring agents – these creams can be used to cover and 'disguise' unwanted colouration of areas of the face.

In this chapter we shall deal with 'coloured' foundation creams.

Coloured foundation creams contain less pigment than cover creams (which will be described below). Therefore, when using foundation creams, the best cosmetic result will be achieved by proper selection of the right shade. This can be obtained by:

- using only foundation creams;
- combining colour correctors with the foundation creams.

If a foundation cream alone is to be used then, when selecting its colour, one should keep in mind that a foundation may appear darker in the container than when it is applied to the skin, because the pigment is in its concentrated form. The undertones of the treated skin should be carefully analyzed and identified in order to achieve the optimal colour matching.

If the foundation cream does not offer adequate coverage, a **colour corrector** can be used. Colour correctors are not foundations. They are designed to be applied under a foundation in order to neutralize light to moderate skin discolouration. In such cases, only after the application of a colour corrector should one use a foundation cream – whose colour should more closely match the skin colour.

Colour correctors are most commonly used to counterbalance ruddiness or sallow undertones of the skin.

When using colour correctors, one should keep in mind some basic principles of proper colour matching:

- Use a green-coloured corrector to conceal and neutralize pink or red skin discolouration.
- Use a lavender-coloured corrector to normalize a sallow shade.
- Use a gold-coloured corrector to tone down grey discolouration.

Applying foundation cream

The foundation should be applied to the skin by lightly spreading it on, using a delicate swab or a disposable sponge (wet or dry), or with the fingertips. This spreads it out more evenly over the skin, and helps it penetrate the skin pores, thereby improving its 'adherence' to the skin so that it remains on the skin for longer. Once applied, the foundation should appear well blended.

What are cover creams?

Cover creams are used to camouflage skin lesions. Basically, they represent a certain subtype of makeup products. They consist of various colouring agents in an oily base.

The colouring agents give the product its covering ability, and in various combinations provide the required colour and appropriate degree of gloss. Substances used for this purpose include various minerals and metal compounds, such as titanium dioxide, iron-based compounds, zinc and magnesium compounds, and other pigments.

Note that in order to be used in camouflaging, there are two important features that characterize cover creams, in comparison with regular makeup products:

- Cover creams should be **opaque**, with superior covering capabilities.
- They should be **stable** on the skin, and should remain on the face for longer than ordinary makeup products. This durability is particularly important when hiding scars. The reason is that the ability of a substance to remain on the skin for a long time depends on its ability to get into the skin pores. A scar does not have any pores, so ordinary makeup would normally not remain on scar tissue for a lengthy period.

Matching cover creams to the skin

It is probably wise to test several different products, from different manufacturers, to find the product with the optimal shade that is most suitable for the

How does the camouflage therapist match the cover creams to the skin?

To successfully match a cover cream to the patient's skin, the camouflage therapist must be able to identify the underlying colours that make up the patient's skin tone. The procedure is performed as follows:

1 The cover cream palette is held by the camouflage therapist alongside the area of skin that is to be camouflaged. The therapist makes a quick scan of each cover cream shade to determine its match to the patient's skin colour.
2 If necessary, a second colour should be added and blended into the cover cream. No more than two cream shades from the cover cream palette should be selected to match the skin tone. The camouflage therapist has to approximate the percentage that will be needed of each of these shades to make the correct colour match.
3 Once the correct shade or shades have been chosen, the camouflage therapist removes a small amount from the container and places it on the back of his/her hand. The cream is rubbed onto the back of his/her hand in a circular motion until it is malleable and spreads easily.
4 Three different colour combinations of no more than two blended colours each are blended and mixed. The formulas are recorded.
5 A small sample of each of the three separate cover cream combinations is applied to the patient's skin.
6 The camouflage therapist examines the patient's face from a distance, trying to choose the best combination of cover cream. The cover cream should meet the edges of the surrounding skin without detection. If the cover cream colour combination is the right shade, it will blend so well (not too light or too dark) that it will barely be noticeable. If the cover cream colour combination is too dark, a little bit more of lighter colour of the two can be added until it matches the patient's skin tone. A pinhead amount of white cover cream can also be used to lighten it up. If it is too light, a little more of a darker shade of the two can be added until the colour of the patient's skin tone is matched as closely as possible.

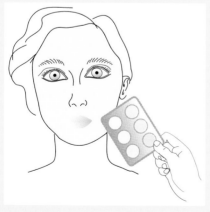

Identifying the underlying colours of the patient's skin.

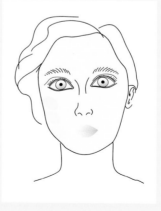

Application of cover cream combinations on the patient's skin.

client. To achieve optimal coverage the makeup should be a little darker than the natural shade of the skin (it should be remembered that the original shade of the makeup changes somewhat once it is applied to the skin, depending on the degree of moisture and the pH of the skin).

In general, it is virtually impossible to attain a perfect colour match. In many cases two products have to be used to achieve the best possible colour. After the right formula has been identified and optimal coverage has been achieved by the camouflage therapist, the patient will be able to regularly perform these camouflage procedures himself/herself.

Applying cover cream

Application of cover cream involves the technique of dabbing on the cream with the third finger (or with a synthetic sponge in a patting motion), rather than rubbing.

The edges of the cover cream should blend well with the surrounding skin to avoid areas of demarcation.

The cover cream layer needs to be stabilized and waterproofed by the application of a colourless powder on its surface to prevent the cover cream from sliding on the skin.

After the problem area has been covered, makeup should be applied to the other side of the face also, in order to achieve a more natural and symmetrical look. Attempts should not be made to cover a lesion or area with the 'perfect' coverage, which may give the face, a strange and unnatural look. It should be remembered that every normal, healthy face has a certain degree of natural imperfection.

Some examples of the use of cover cream are shown below.

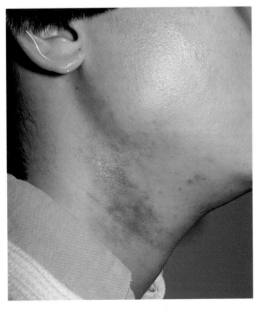 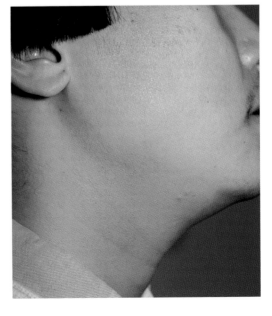

Camouflage of a hyperpigmented scar.

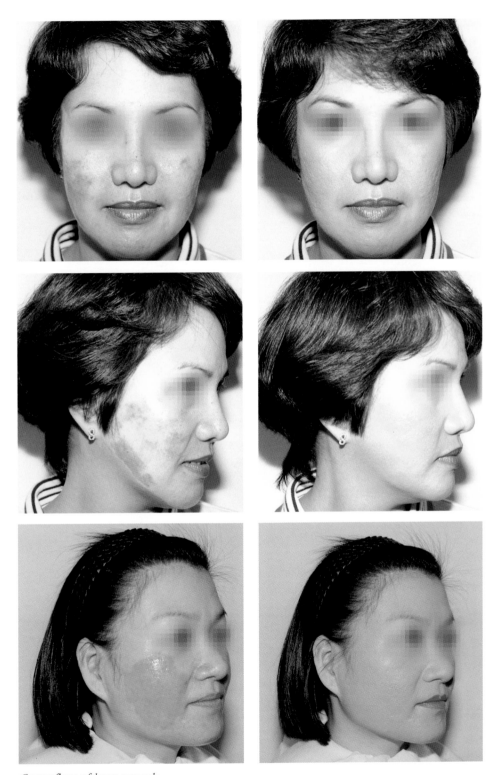

Camouflage of burn wounds.

Determining the right application method for the three distinct types of skin

There are three distinct types of skin with regard to the level of moisture: dry, oily and normal. Each requires a different cover cream application method to ensure the best result.

Dry skin
If the skin is dehydrated and dry in texture, the cover cream should be applied, and left to remain on the skin before being set with powder for up to ten minutes, and then a colourless powder should be applied and quickly brushed off to prevent the area from looking scaly.

Oily skin
The cover cream should be applied and powdered, and the talc should be left sitting on top of the cover cream mixture for up to ten minutes to absorb the oils in the product before the powder is brushed off.

Normal skin
The cover cream should be applied and powdered, and the powder should be brushed off immediately to produce the most natural effect.

Recreating skin imperfections

In certain instances, to provide the most natural cosmetic result, one must recreate the appearance of imperfections on the skin. Freckles, beard stubble and broken veins can all be reproduced with the use of cosmetic sponges. To stipple-in freckles, broken veins or beard stubble over a comestic camouflaged area, one would simply press a wedge-type cosmetic sponge into a cover cream mixture. To determine the amount of pressure required to imitate the skin irregularity, the sponge should be pressed down on the back of one's hand before applying it to the skin area. Using the stipple sponge as an applicator, powder is afterwards applied to set and waterproof the application. To reproduce broken capillaries, a rose cover cream can be used, to imitate freckles a golden-brown mixture can be used, while for beard stubble one should select (depending on the beard colour) a brown, dark brown, grey or black cover cream.

25

Structure of hair and principles of hair care

Contents Overview • Definition: hair follicle • Types of hair • How many hair follicles are there? • Structure of hair • Transverse section of the hair shaft • Life cycle of the hair • Rate of hair growth • Hair care: which manipulations affect hair growth? • Hair loss and baldness

Overview

The social, psychological, and sexual significance of the scalp and body hair is immense. Any change in the pattern of the hair – too much hair, too little hair, change of colour – may have far-reaching emotional consequences for the person involved. However, the remainder of this chapter will not discuss the social and sexual significance of hair. Rather, it will deal with general facts about the scalp and body hair and general suggestions regarding hair care: how best to care for the scalp hair.

Definition: hair follicle

The hair follicle is an elongated tube-like structure in the skin. It is lined by cells, and the hair grows out of the base of the follicle.

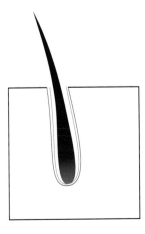

Schematic representation of a hair follicle.

Types of hair

Vellus hair
This is fine, short, light-coloured hair. Its length rarely exceeds two centimetres.

Terminal hair
Terminal hair is longer, thicker, more pigmented, coarser and stiffer than vellus hair. Before adolescence terminal hair is found only on the scalp, the eyebrows and the eyelashes. During sexual maturation, in response to hormonal changes, some hair follicles from which vellus hair previously grew start to produce terminal hair.

Intermediate type
Apart from the two types of hair noted above, there are some hairs that represent an intermediate form. These are somewhere in the wide range between the vellus hair type and the terminal hair type.

How many hair follicles are there?

The average number of hair follicles on a person's body surface is approximately five million. There is no significant difference in the number of hair follicles between men and women, or between different races. The differences in the appearance of hair between men and women are due to the type of hair produced by a follicle. Hair follicles do not develop after birth.

Some regions of the body have no hair follicles: the palms and soles, the red parts of the lips, the umbilicus, the nipples, the skin over the joints of the fingers and toes, and parts of the genitalia. All the other apparently hairless parts of the body are, in fact, covered with fine, almost invisible, vellus hair.

> ### Number of hair follicles on the scalp
>
> The average number of hair follicles on the scalp is approximately 100 000. This figure is an average, and applies to people with dark hair. The number varies, depending on hereditary factors and the shade of hair. Redheads have relatively less, but thicker, scalp hair (the average is 80 000). People with blond hair have thinner hair, but more of it – approximately 120 000 hair follicles on the scalp.
>
> With age there is a gradual loss of hair follicles from the scalp, to varying degrees.

Structure of hair

The hair consists of an elongated part, which grows from the dermis and protrudes above the surface of the skin, known as the **hair shaft**. Hair grows

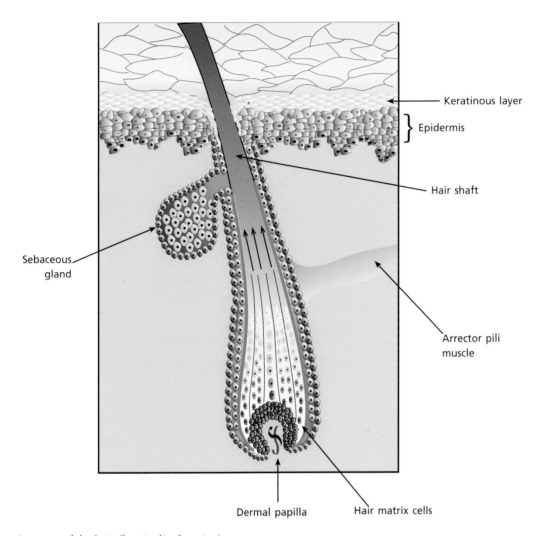

Structure of the hair (longitudinal section).

from a **hair follicle** – an elongated tubular structure in the skin, which is lined with cells. One or more **sebaceous glands** open into the hair follicle. A fatty substance called **sebum** is produced by the sebaceous glands, and passes via a short duct from the gland into the hair follicle. An **arrector pili muscle** is attached to the hair follicle; when this muscle contracts, it causes the hair to stand up. As can be seen from the diagram, the bottom of the follicle is wider and thicker. The region below the lower end of the follicle is called the **papilla**. It is also called the **dermal** or **follicular papilla**; it contains blood vessels that nourish the hair follicle.

At the bottom of the hair follicle are the unique cells that produce the hair itself. These cells have enormous replicating abilities. They divide, and as more and more cells appear, the older ones are 'pushed' upward in vertical rows and gradually degenerate. Since the cells degenerate and die as they move up the follicle, the upper part of the hair is made up of dead cells, which remain attached to each other by an intercellular cement-like substance. In other words, the hair that protrudes above the skin is actually made of dead keratinous (horny) material. The only living part of the hair is the cells at the bottom of the hair at the base of the hair follicle, which constantly divide, and determine the hair quality.

As long as the cells at the bottom of the hair follicle (which form the base of the hair) are healthy and normal, the hair can continue growing. If, for any reason, those cells are destroyed, there will no longer be any hair growing from that follicle.

Hair formation

The process by which hair is formed resembles the way in which the keratinous (horny) layer of the skin forms. The cells at the base of both the epidermis and the hair follicle divide and then are pushed upward, degenerate and die. In the course of this process of degeneration, cells accumulate large amounts of a protein called **keratin**. This is, in fact, the major component of the keratinous (horny) layer of the skin. Keratin imparts to the outer layer of the skin its horn-like consistency (it is the substance from which horns of mammals are mainly built).

In hair follicles, the cells produce a different keratinous substance. – another protein of especially hard consistency, called 'hard keratin', which is chemically different from the usual keratin of the skin.

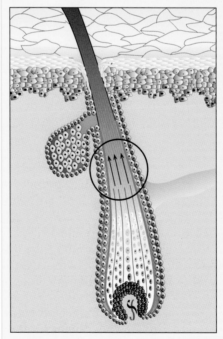

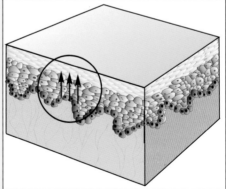

Formation of hair.   *Formation of the keratinous layer of the skin.*

Hair colour

In the same way that the **melanocytes** (**melanin**-producing cells) in the skin give it its colour, the melanocytes in the hair follicle give the hair its specific colour. Different types of melanin, which differ from one person to another according to each one's genetic characteristics, determine the hair's final colour. Different concentrations and different chemical compositions of melanin produce blond, brown or black hair.

- A compound called **eumelanin** makes a hair brown–black; when the concentration of eumelanin is relatively low, the hair is blond.
- A compound called **pheomelanin** imparts a red colour to the hair.
- When the hair loses its pigment, it becomes grey or white.

Microscopic structure of hair shaft

The major component of hair is the protein keratin. The hair shaft is made up of many thin fibres of keratin twisted together into thicker bundles, as shown below.

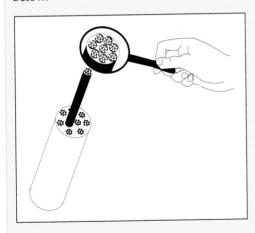

Microscopic structure of the hair shaft: thin fibres linked into thicker bundles.

Transverse section of the hair shaft

The hair shaft is made up of three layers:

- the **medulla**
- the **cortex**
- the **cuticle**

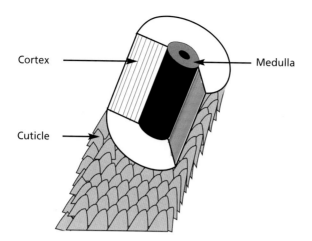

Transverse section of the hair shaft.

Cortex

Medulla

Cuticle

Cortex

This is the central layer; it is made up of hair cells that are constantly moving upward, and as they do so they degenerate and die. The cells are connected to each other by a cement-like substance.

Cuticle

This lies outside the cortex, and is a sort of thin outer wrapping. This layer is made up of cells that partially overlap, as shown in the diagram. The cuticle is relatively impermeable, and protects the hair from penetration of foreign materials.

If the cuticular layer is intact, and the cells overlap each other in an orderly fashion (as they are meant to), the hair looks soft and shiny, since light rays are reflected from it evenly. On the other hand, if the cuticle is damaged (for example, by incorrect treatment of hair, such as by excessive brushing, waving, straightening or dyeing), the cuticular layer loses its uniformity, the hair loses its sheen, and the ends of the hair become frayed and split.

Medulla

This is a thin layer in the centre of the hair shaft. Sometimes the medulla is absent, or is not continuous along the length of the hair. Its presence or absence may affect the sheen and colouring of the hair.

Life cycle of the hair

Every hair follicle has a regular life cycle, of growth, rest, and falling out. The cycle of any single hair is not dependent on the others – there is no synchronization. Therefore it is normal and natural for up to one hundred scalp hairs to be shed daily and about one hundred other hairs will appear in their place.

Some of the complaints of hair loss that are brought to the doctor merely reflect this normal cycle. In such cases, obviously no medical treatment is necessary, other than reassurance and explaining to the patient that this shedding of hair is a well-recognized phenomenon and is quite normal.

Stages in the life cycle of the hair

Anagen: the active growing phase
In anagen, the hair cells at the base of the hair follicle are dividing repeatedly, and the hair grows steadily. This growth phase can last from several months to several years (on the scalp, the average time is approximately three years). The length of this phase determines the maximum length that the hair will reach, and it varies from person to person.

Catagen: the transition phase
This relatively brief phase, lasting some two to four weeks, is a transitional phase during which the hair stops growing.

Telogen: the resting phase
Telogen lasts three to six months. During this period, the mechanism responsible for the replication of the cells at the base of the hair, and the subsequent hair growth, are inactive for several months. By the end of telogen, the hair is only loosely attached to the follicle, and can be easily pulled out simply by brushing or washing the hair, etc. It is hairs in this phase that come away readily from the scalp when pulled.

Resumption of active growth
After the resting phase, a new hair will appear from the same follicle during the next anagen (growth) phase. As this new hair grows, it pushes the old one, which is shed from the follicle.

Normally, at any given time, approximately 80–90% of the hairs on the head are in the anagen (growth) phase, and 10–15% are in the telogen (resting) phase. Less than 1% are in the catagen phase. As noted above, the cycles of the different hair follicles are in no way related to each other. Hence, in a normal scalp, the normal shedding of the hairs in the telogen phase is not noticeable.

The duration of the various phases of the cycle differs in different parts of the body. For example, scalp hair has different cycle periods to those of body hair.

Life cycle of a hair

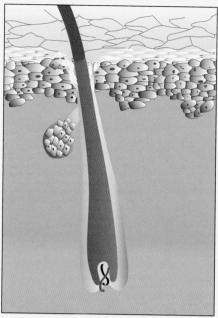

1 Active growth phase (anagen): cells at the base of the hair follicle divide repeatedly, and the hair grows steadily.

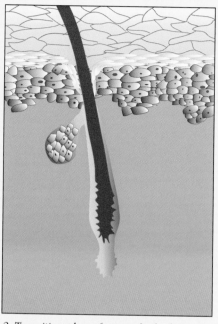

2 Transition phase (catagen): the hair follicle becomes shorter.

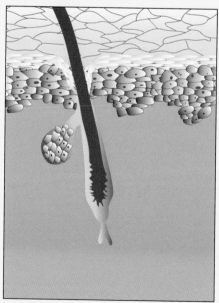

3 Resting phase (telogen): cells at the base of the hair follicle are not dividing; the hair is shorter, located more superficially – nearer to the skin surface.

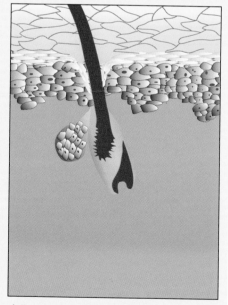

4 Resumption of the growth phase (new anagen phase): from the same follicle, from a growth centre lower down (compared with the 'old' hair), a new hair starts to grow.

Normal and abnormal hair loss

The hairs that normally fall out are in the **telogen** phase. A telogen hair is club-shaped – i.e. a thin shaft, with a wider 'blob' at the base. As opposed to anagen hair, its base is devoid of pigment. This can be seen clearly with a magnifying glass or microscope.

Because telogen hairs have this shape, people tend to mistakenly think that the hair has come out 'with the root', and that a new hair will not grow in its place. In fact, just the opposite is true: a club-shaped hair that has fallen out is normal, and is a manifestation of the natural and reasonable shedding of up to 100 telogen hairs each day. **If that is the case, then how can a doctor tell for certain when hair loss is normal and when it is abnormal?**

The signs of abnormal hair loss are as follows:

- When more than 100 telogen hairs are shed in a day.
- When the hair starts to visibly thin out.
- The hairs that are shed are not telogen hairs. Certain medical problems may lead to this abnormal status. A dermatologist can identify this abnormality by examining the shed hairs.

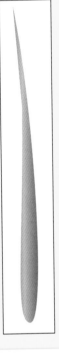

A telogen hair.

Rate of hair growth

Scalp hair grows at a rate of up to 0.4 mm a day during a growth period of three to five years; its average length is 70 cm, but it can grow up to 100 cm. Body hair grows at a slower rate than scalp hair, at 0.2 mm per day, and the growth period is two to six months. These hairs ultimately reach a length of 1–3 cm.

Both the period of active growth, and the rate of growth, vary from person to person. Largely hereditary factors determine the length of the growth period and rate of growth. The length of the growth period and the rate of growth also vary with age. They differ between males and females – body hair of women grows more slowly than that of men, whereas scalp hair grows faster in women than in men. Nutritional, hormonal and other constitutional factors also affect hair growth.

A fast growth rate and relatively long growth period are determined genetically, which explains why some women's hair is particularly long, while other women's hair never grows beyond shoulder length, even if they do not cut it.

Hair care: which manipulations affect hair growth?

Factors that may affect hair growth include:

- pulling or stretching the hair
- local pressure on the scalp
- certain externally applied substances
- local heat

Pulling or stretching the hair

Cutting the hair has no effect on growth, which takes place at the bottom of the hair follicle. On the other hand, pulling the hair and exerting some tension on the root could cause damage to the root, weakening it, and making the hair shed more readily.

Tension on the hair can occur as a result of combing the hair back and fastening it tightly with a clip or pin. Loss of hair in this way is usually apparent at the temples or the forehead, because that is where the hair is under the maximal tension. A similar phenomenon can occur following the use of hair rollers.

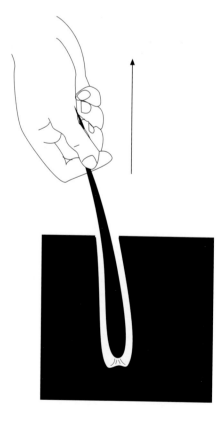

Pulling on the hair applies tension to the root and may damage it.

Similarly, curly hair can be pulled and possibly damaged by being combed in the opposite direction to its natural growth.

In addition:

- over-vigorous brushing;
- over-vigorous massaging and rubbing of the scalp and hair when washing it;
- drying the hair by rubbing it too vigorously (the correct way to dry hair is to absorb the water by gently patting the head with the towel).

With time, any of the above can cause damage to the hair and increase hair loss. If someone already has a tendency to hair loss, he/she should take particular care to wash the hair gently and dry it by gentle patting, to minimize the already existing damage.

Local pressure on the scalp

This is a relatively uncommon problem, which is probably caused by interference with the local blood supply to the scalp. In infants who sleep on their backs, a bald area often appears at the back of the head. An identical phenomenon may be seen after some major surgical operations, following which patients lie on their backs without moving for long periods.

Externally applied substances

Many externally applied products on the cosmetic market claim to 'revive' hair roots by supplying basic 'building' materials and in that way encourage and accelerate hair growth and prevent hair loss. Most of those substances do not even reach the hair root, nor are they absorbed into the root, which is located deep in the dermis. There is no proof that these products have any effect on hair growth. (A medication that *has* been shown to affect and accelerate – to a certain extent – hair growth following its local application is a substance called **minoxidil**.)

On the other hand, certain toxic substances, whether absorbed into the body or applied locally, may damage the hair follicles. Therefore care should be taken when selecting a product for dyeing, straightening or curling the hair, and to ensure that it is produced by a reputable, recognized cosmetics manufacturer.

Among the numerous depilatory products available on the market for removing excess hair, there are substances that can dissolve the keratinous (horny) substance of which the hair is made. These products have no effect on the living part of the hair. (This is discussed in more detail in Chapter 28 on methods of temporary removal of hair.)

Local heat

Heating of the scalp usually occurs as a result of using equipment to dry, curl or straighten hair (electric rollers or hair 'irons'). A shower that is too hot and vigorous also does not benefit the hair. The resultant high temperatures near the hair root can cause damage.

Hair loss and baldness

Apart from what has previously been said in this chapter, we shall not deal with hair loss and baldness other than to state the following: **The investigation of hair loss and baldness should be performed only by a physician.**

Apart from the common male baldness, there are many possible causes of hair loss and baldness in men and women, such as hormonal factors, dietary deficiencies (of various vitamins or iron), exposure to toxic substances, infections, and other diseases.

This is not a problem that cosmeticians should attempt to manage. The best thing that a cosmetician can do when asked about a hair loss problem is to refer the client to a dermatologist.

26

Shampoo

Contents Washing hair: overview • Surfactants • The best shampoo •
Components of shampoo • Dandruff and anti-dandruff preparations •
'Gentle' shampoos • Washing the hair • Appendix: details of shampoo
ingredients

Note: It is recommended that this chapter be read after reading Chapter 5 on
skin cleansing.

Washing hair: overview

The scalp and hair are normally lubricated by sebum, which is secreted from
the sebaceous glands. This oily secretion protects the hair and skin against
water loss, and gives the hair its sheen. On the other hand, there is some disadvantage to the oily layer on the scalp – dust, soot, and other environmental
pollutants tend to stick to it, as do particles of keratin from the skin.

The same principle that applies to cleansing the skin also applies to sham-
pooing hair: in order to remove the dust, soot, and other grime, as well as the
cells of the keratin layer that have peeled off, **the oily layer on the scalp and
hair must be removed, since these particles are embedded in it.** In addition,
the same principle that applies to the action of soaps and surfactants for
cleansing the skin also applies to shampoos for cleaning the scalp and hair.
The surfactants, the active ingredients in shampoos, surround and trap tiny
droplets of fat (that contain the grime), and these are removed from the scalp
and hair by rinsing with water.

Why should one not use normal soap?

Normal soap has two major drawbacks, so it is not recommended for washing the
hair:

- Normal soap has a high pH, which damages skin and hair.
- The use of normal soap with tap water produces calcium salts that adhere to
  the hair. This causes the hair to feel 'fragile', look dull, and be dishevelled and
  hard to comb.

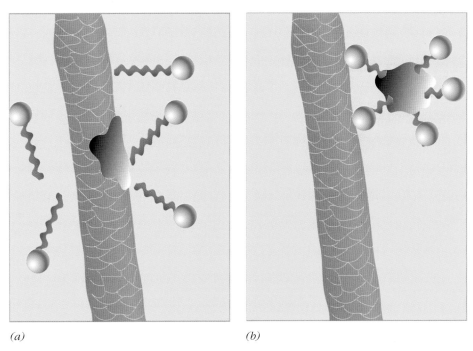

(a)   (b)

The principle of action of shampoo is identical to that of soap: (a) a particle of fat and grime adherent to a hair shaft; (b) surfactants trap the fat particle and remove it from the hair.

Shampoos are designed to replace ordinary soap. The basic compounds within shampoos are surfactants.

Surfactants

Surfactants (surface-active agents), which are water-soluble compounds, constitute the major component of soaps and shampoos. Surfactants clean by virtue of their chemical structure. They 'surround' the fat, with its embedded grime, by forming chemical structures called micelles, so that on rinsing with water, the fat and dirt can be removed from the hair or skin. There are four main groups of surfactants, distinguished from each other by their chemical structure and electric charge:

- anionic surfactants
- cationic surfactants
- non-ionic surfactants
- amphoteric surfactants

Different surfactants have different properties, and vary in their abilities to clean, create a lather, and impart lustre or softness to hair. Shampoos usually do not contain just one surfactant, but a combination of several, designed for use on different types of hair. For example, anionic surfactants have good cleaning properties. Therefore anionic surfactants are commonly found in most shampoos. On the labels of most shampoos will be found the names **sodium lauryl sulfate** and **sodium laureth sulfate**, which are anionic surfactants.

Natural surfactants

These are another type of surfactant. They are made up of saponins, which are derived from various plants. Saponins are good at creating foam, but less effective at cleaning. They are therefore usually used in combination with the usual synthetic surfactants to achieve effective cleaning and good cosmetic results.

The best shampoo

As noted above, a shampoo is not meant only to clean, but will fulfil several other functions, in accordance with the demands of the customer. A shampoo should be adapted to the individual in terms of the following aspects:

Hair type
- Is the hair dry or oily?
- Is the hair thin?
- Has the hair been bleached, dyed or waved?

Specific scalp problems
For example, does the user have dandruff?

Safety requirements
- Does the preparation irritate the eyes?
- Does the preparation irritate the scalp?

Personal preferences of the user
These may include the following:

- the shampoo's consistency and texture (a shampoo may be in the form of a liquid or a cream);
- the presence of a particular fragrance;
- the ease and convenience of application of the shampoo;
- the ease with which it spreads through the hair;
- the amount of foam it produces, and its quality and texture;
- how easy it is to rinse off;
- the degree to which it makes the hair soft, supple and shiny;
- how easy it is to comb and manage the hair after using the shampoo.

Similarly, the shampoo should be appropriate for the season of the year, for the frequency of use, and for other specific demands of the consumer.

Components of shampoo

Up to this point, we have confined our discussion to the role of surfactants in cleaning hair. However, if a shampoo were to contain only cleansing agents whose task it was to remove the fatty layer from the hair and scalp, the hair would end up becoming dull, coarse, and hard to comb and manage.

What other constituents are there in shampoo that make it more acceptable to the user?

1 A mixture of several surfactants is needed. A single surfactant usually cannot guarantee that a shampoo will achieve what is required. Note that some surfactants have properties other than simply cleaning. Some have good foaming capabilities, as well as being effective in conditioning and softening the hair.
2 Moisturizers – as needed, when the hair tends to be dry.
3 Conditioners.
4 Foaming agents.
5 Water softeners (chelating agents).
6 Thickeners.
7 Pearlescents.
8 Coloring agents.
9 Perfumes.
10 Preservatives.
11 'Special' ingredients.

Surfactants
The role of surfactants has been discussed above.

Moisturizers
In many cases, moisturizing agents have to be added to the shampoo, because cleansing with a surfactant results in the removal of the natural oil. Without oil, the hair becomes dull and loses its softness, which makes it hard to comb and manage. The hair becomes more fragile, and tends to split at the ends. This phenomenon of dry hair is usually the result of several factors: dry weather, exposure to wind, air pollution, swimming pools containing chlorine, and the use of 'hard' shampoos that dry the hair. These characteristics are even more pronounced in hair that has been bleached or dyed. Shampoo removes the unwanted oil and grime from the hair and scalp, but it also removes the oil that the hair needs, which gives it lustre and softness.

Therefore shampoo should be tailored to the particular type of hair: someone with oily hair requires a shampoo that is more effective in removing oil, while someone with dry hair requires a shampoo with a less vigorous, gentler cleaning effect, and with added moisturizer.

In general, tailoring the shampoo to the user in terms of the amount of moisturizer it contains should be related to the type of skin on the scalp: if the scalp is dry, the hair tends to be dry, with an oily scalp, the hair also tends to be oily.

Conditioners

The purpose of conditioners is to make the hair soft, shiny, and easier to comb and manage. Conditioners are a particularly important component of shampoos used for dry or damaged hair (following colouring, waving, etc.).

In general, many dermatologists advise using a conditioner after washing the hair with shampoo, rather than using a shampoo that contains a conditioner. This is because two different functions are involved here: cleansing and conditioning. A shampoo that contains conditioner has to fulfil several functions, the chief being cleansing the hair. Such a shampoo cannot achieve the efficiency of a pure conditioner, used independently, after washing and cleaning the hair. Furthermore, remnants of shampoo that remain on the hair after using a conditioner-containing shampoo must obviously contain cleansing agents – and should be avoided.

Hair conditioners are discussed in more detail in Chapter 27.

Other components

These include foaming agents, chelating agents, thickeners, pearlescents, dyes, fragrances and preservatives.

Foaming agents

These act by producing bubbles in the water, creating a lather. Note that there are many shampoos that clean effectively without producing lather. However, the inclusion of foaming agents in shampoos may be seen as an advantage from the marketing point of view, since the current public opinion seems to associate a lather with efficient cleaning. In fact, there is no need for an extensive lather to clean effectively: the effectiveness of a shampoo is mainly determined by how the hair looks and how the user feels after washing the hair, and not by how much lather it produces.

Water softeners (chelating or sequestering agents)

These bind ('chelate') calcium and magnesium ions present in water, and thereby prevent their attachment to fatty acids, which would create salts that are not easily soluble. Without the addition of water softeners, the salts that form would affect the cleansing ability by coating the hair. This coating stays on the hair as a thin layer, and makes the hair lose its lustre.

Thickeners

These make the shampoo thicker. Thickeners have nothing to do with the cleansing properties of the shampoo. However, they make the shampoo look more attractive. Apart from that, people tend to think that the thicker a shampoo, the more effective it is, and the 'richer in active ingredients'. This is by no means true, and the consistency of a shampoo is not necessarily related to its effectiveness. Nevertheless, there is some advantage to a shampoo that is thicker in consistency, in that a thicker shampoo is less likely to dribble down and get into the user's eyes.

Pearlescents

These are added to shampoos to change their appearance and give them a 'pearly' sheen.

Dyes and perfumes

The reason for using dyes or perfumes is obvious. However, it is preferable not to use shampoos that incorporate synthetic dyes, or perfumes that are particularly strong. These may irritate the scalp, cause allergic reactions, or even damage the outer layers of the hair.

Preservatives

Other substances are incorporated into shampoos to preserve them:

- various preservatives;
- anti-oxidants;
- emulsifiers, whose task it is to stabilize the mixture of ingredients that make up the shampoo (some surfactants also act as emulsifiers).

'Special' ingredients in shampoo

These substances may include various vitamins (e.g. vitamins B and E), plant extracts, egg, honey, jojoba, aloe vera, and others. The shampoo industry creates a whimsical and crowded market, and the use of these ingredients may have significant effects on sales, especially if some particular ingredient happens to be 'in vogue' at the time.

At present, most interest is centred around substances from the vitamin B group (particularly vitamin B_5 and B_6). Cosmetics and pharmaceutical companies report that the regular use of substances containing these vitamins 'strengthens' the hair, moisturizes it, and gives the hair a healthy sheen. They claim that the hair becomes more supple, and less fragile. However, there are no reports in the scientific literature or studies that support these contentions, and these claims have not yet been tested by accepted scientific criteria.

With regard to the use of these substances, it should be remembered that **the hair shaft is made of dead keratin. The external hair cannot be 'nourished', nor can its growth be influenced by something applied to this keratinous material.**

Nevertheless, what can these substances do?

Applying them to the external hair can affect its appearance (but not its growth!). The hair will look shinier and 'silkier', and will be easier to comb and manage. If, then, shampoos that contain these special ingredients may have some advantage over standard shampoos, in terms of the appearance and manageability of the hair, their use is basically up to the user's personal preference. It is reasonable to assume that, in many cases, users will prefer these preparations. After all, cosmetics manufacturers spend a fortune to try and convince people to use their product.

Do these substances penetrate the living tissue – the hair root – and affect hair growth?

For most of the 'exotic' ingredients, this has never been proven. In any case, if a substance is to have some effect on the hair root, it is better applied to the hair in the form of a solution, which will remain there for several hours, rather than as a component of a shampoo. In the case of a shampoo, any component will be in contact with the scalp for a very short time only, and most of it ends up going down the drain, together with the shampoo and water.

Dandruff and anti-dandruff preparations

Although dandruff is not a disease or a serious problem, it is disturbing to the sufferer, and poses an aesthetic nuisance. Dandruff is common – about 80% of the population has dandruff at some stage in their lives, mainly between the ages of 20 and 40. Because it is so common, one can think of it to some extent as being a normal phenomenon, so long as it is not excessive or becomes a nuisance.

What is dandruff?

Dandruff is, in effect, particles of keratin that are shed from the skin. There is a constant turnover of epidermal cells in the skin. At the base of the epidermis, new cells are constantly being formed, and migrate to the surface, where they are eventually shed. As long as the rate of this turnover is reasonable and normal, it is hard to actually see the shed cells. If, however, the rate of turnover increases, more and more dead keratinous cells are produced, which adhere to particles of keratin, and become visible to the naked eye as they are shed from the skin.

Dandruff can appear in normal (neither dry nor oily) hair. Sometimes, if the scalp is particularly dry, and the dry skin peels, this can look like dandruff. Nevertheless, dandruff is more common in oily hair.

Most dandruff scales are grey–white in colour, but if the scalp is very oily then larger scales are formed, which are oily and have a yellowish colour.

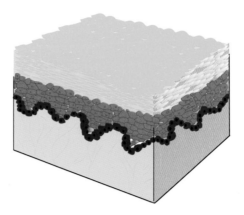

Microscopic appearance of the skin covered by a layer of dandruff scales.

Seborrhoea and seborrhoeic dermatitis

- In **seborrhoea** the sebaceous glands are overactive, producing an excess of sebum. The hair looks oily. This is usually associated with dandruff.
- **Seborrhoeic dermatitis** is a chronic skin inflammation that occurs in areas with extensive sebaceous glands. In adults, it tends to appear in the scalp, face and upper trunk. In seborrhoeic dermatitis, the affected areas of skin are red, and covered by oily scales.
- **Cradle cap** is a severe form of seborrhoeic dermatitis in infants, which looks like a greasy, scaly layer on the baby's scalp.

See further page 138.

What causes dandruff?

This subject is still somewhat controversial, but most researchers see dandruff as a mild form of seborrhoeic dermatitis. The exact reason for the appearance of dandruff is, however, not clear. Hereditary and hormonal factors also seem to be involved. There is a seasonal effect, with the problem tending to be worse in the winter months. There is also a tendency for dandruff to be aggravated by emotional stress or a physical ailment (such as a febrile illness).

It has been suggested that dandruff (and seborrhoeic dermatitis) are associated with the presence of a microscopic yeast called **Pityrosporum ovale** on the scales and in the hair follicles. Some shampoos designed for treating dandruff contain substances aimed at eradicating this yeast from the scalp.

In the same way that different shampoos are based on variations of the same basic constituents (surfactants), with each manufacturer producing its particular combinations of constituents, so also with shampoos for the treatment of dandruff.

The same basic ingredients appear in various combinations in virtually all anti-dandruff shampoos – one can see this by reading the labels. The fact is that no cosmetics or pharmaceutical manufacturer has 'invented the wheel', and no-one has developed the ultimate anti-dandruff shampoo.

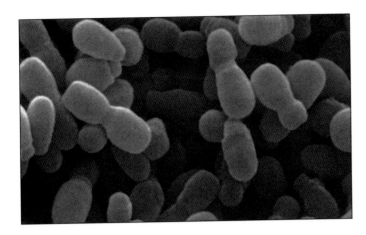

Pityrosporum ovale *visualized by scanning electron microscopy.*

The guiding principle in the treatment of dandruff, as far as the consumer is concerned, is that if a shampoo of a given type has not helped, one can switch to a shampoo of a different type. In most cases, one will eventually find a shampoo that does achieve a definite improvement.

Anti-dandruff ingredients in various shampoos

Zinc pyrithione and pyridine derivatives

These substances slow down the rapid cell turnover – slowing down the turnover rate of epidermal cells means that fewer scales are produced. Furthermore, these substances are effective against *Pityrosporum ovale*, which is now considered, if not the cause, at least an additional factor in the development of dandruff. They are present in many non-prescription shampoos.

Quaternary ammonium surfactants

These compounds belong to the cationic surfactant group. They have antibacterial and antifungal effects. In addition, they decrease the production of free fatty acids, which are the cause of the irritant effect of sebum, so they have a soothing effect.

Sulfur derivatives, including selenium disulfide

The main effect of these substances is **keratolytic**, i.e. they dissolve the keratinous of the keratin layer of the skin, thereby preventing the formation of visible flakes of keratin. In addition, they also slow down the rate of turnover of the epidermal cells. Sulfur derivatives are best used for short periods of treatment, since they may result in breaking of the hair shafts.

Tar

It is not clear how tar works in the treatment of dandruff, but it is probably related mainly to the slowing down of epidermal cell turnover. Hence products based on tar are also useful in other inflammatory skin conditions, such as psoriasis, in which there is excessive cell turnover. Tar also has a degree of antiseptic activity, and is also antipruritic (prevents itching). The medical ramifications of using tar in shampoo for long periods are controversial. Usually, these products are well tolerated. However, the European Community has decided recently that tar products should be removed from the market.

Piroctone olamine
This substance decreases dandruff by slowing down epidermal cell turnover. It is also claimed to be effective against *Pityrosporum ovale*.

Antifungal medications
These medications act directly on the microscopic yeast *Pityrosporum ovale*. Because they contain antifungal medications, some are available only on a doctor's prescription. Shampoo preparations containing antifungal medications may eliminate production of dandruff in cases where non-prescription shampoo preparations did not show any beneficial effect. Since they contain an active medication, some should only be used for a limited period. The usual recommendation is to wash the hair twice a week for up to a month, and no more. Such a course of treatment should be sufficient to eliminate the yeast and prevent dandruff.

Use of anti-dandruff shampoos
To obtain the best results from any anti-dandruff shampoo, the shampoo should be left on the scalp for about three to five minutes, or according to the manufacturer's instructions, and then rinsed off. If the preparation is in contact with the scalp for a shorter period, its effect will be reduced.

In more severe cases, when there is no improvement with the above shampoos, a dermatologist should be consulted. The dermatologist may advise applying an oily preparation containing **salicylic acid** to the scalp for a number of hours before rinsing. Salicylic acid dissolves the scales attached to the scalp.

In cases of seborrhoeic dermatitis, a dermatologist must be consulted.

'Gentle' shampoos

So-called 'gentle' shampoos are shampoos for people with delicate skin, or more particularly, for babies. They also are designed not to cause stinging of the eyes, which results from certain ingredients in shampoos getting into the eyes. The special nature of these preparations is based on the following:

- They are supposed not to contain ingredients that may cause irritation, particularly perfumes and certain preservatives.
- Many contain a relatively higher concentration of **betaines**, which are surfactants from the amphoteric group. These surfactants are relatively gentle, and do not tend to cause skin or eye irritation.

Washing the hair

Method of washing

Hair is composed largely of dead keratinous material. Thus, for example, cutting a hair, which is dead keratin, has no effect on the active cells at the base of the hair follicle, and can have no effect on the growth or vitality of the hair. However, pulling the hair can affect the root. Hence, when applying shampoo, this should be done gently and not roughly, and there is no need to massage the hair or scalp vigorously when washing it. By the same token, the hair should be dried gently and not roughly.

People with sparse or thin hair should be even more gentle when drying their hair, and it should be patted dry rather than rubbed.

When washing hair, very hot water should not be used, since repeated use of water that is too hot can damage the hair.

Shampoo should be kept away from the eyes – even the 'gentle' shampoos that usually do not cause eye irritation. Every last bit of shampoo should be washed out of the hair, since shampoo remaining on the scalp may cause skin irritation. Therefore it is advisable to rinse the hair for three to four minutes after washing it.

Recommended frequency of washing

There is no specific recommended frequency for washing hair. Each person has his/her optimal time scale, depending on whether the hair is dry or oily, how much physical exercise the person engages in, their occupation, and their degree of exposure to dust, soot and other environmental pollutants. People with oily hair, particularly if they are exposed to dirt, soot, etc. during the day, may need to wash their hair daily. If the hair is gently washed, there is no reason for avoiding a daily shampoo.

Appendix: details of shampoo ingredients

Moisturizers are discussed in Chapter 4.

Conditioners are discussed in Chapter 27.

Foaming agents: the main substances used for this purpose are **fatty acid alkanoamides**, which produce a soft lather, as well as various surfactants that are able to produce a lather.

Water softeners: the most widely used are EDTA and citric acid.

Thickeners: the most widely used substances are 'natural' gums (such as tragacanth and karaya), hydrocolloid substances, acrylic polymers (such as carbomer), and salts such as sodium and ammonium chloride.

Pearlescents: the most commonly used substances are **alcohol sulfates** and **fatty acid esters.**

Dyes, fragrances, and preservatives are discussed in Chapter 3 on the principles of preparation of medical and cosmetic products.

27

Hair conditioners

Contents Overview • What happens if the outer surface of a hair is damaged? • What activities damage hair? • The principle behind the action of a hair conditioner • Types of hair conditioner • How to use a hair conditioner • Frequency of use of a hair conditioner • Hair styling: hair mousses and hair gels

Overview

The **cuticle** is the outer layer of the hair shaft (see Chapter 25 on the structure of hair). Its integrity and health determine the appearance of scalp hair. The properties of hair, such as its softness, lustre and pliability, are determined mainly by what happens on its surface. Hair conditioners treat the external surface of the hair.

What happens if the outer surface of a hair is damaged?

The lustre of hair is the result of the light reflecting off each individual hair. If there is damage to the surface of the hair, there is less reflection of light, and the hair loses its shine and lustre.

If the external surface of the hair is damaged, the hair shaft develops negative electrostatic charges along its length. As a result of the electrical charge, the hairs repel each other, which makes it very difficult to comb or manage the hair.

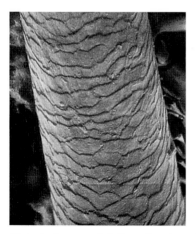 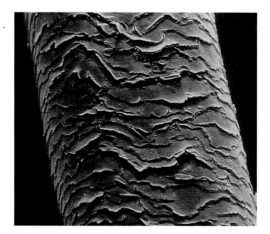

Hair shaft: normal (left) and with early signs of damage (right), as shown by a scanning electron microscope.

The smoothness and softness of a hair are thought to be related to the orderly and uniform arrangement of the cuticle. A normal, healthy cuticle looks like the arrangement of roof tiles. Should the cuticle be damaged, the surface of the hair shaft becomes irregular and disorganized, and the hair becomes rougher and coarser. The hair becomes more brittle, and the ends tend to fray and split.

What activities damage hair?

Hair can be damaged by the following:

- washing the hair too frequently (however, if the hair is short and the shampoo is mild, there is only minimal damage);
- too frequent combing and brushing;
- overuse of a hair dryer;
- waving;
- dyeing with permanent dyes;
- bleaching the hair;
- exposure to certain environmental conditions, such as the sun's radiation, wind and swimming pool water.

All of the above activities damage the cuticle of the hair shaft. As a result, the hair becomes rough, loses its lustre, becomes stiff and fragile, and is harder to comb and arrange.

Note: The above list refers to agents or activities that affect the external hair, that which is above the surface of the skin, by damaging the external surface of the hair – the cuticle. This means that all of these agents damage the dead keratinous layer of the hair shaft, but usually have no effect on the hair cells deep inside the hair follicle. Hence they *usually* have no effect on the growth of the hair, so that after exposure to the above damaging agents, as the hair grows out, it will gradually regain its original, healthy appearance.

Nevertheless, if the above activities are exaggerated and excessive, some damage may occur to the living cells inside the follicle, which will affect hair growth. For example, excessive use of a hair dryer can result in heating up of the area, which can damage the living cells in the hair follicle. Activities that tend to pull on the hair, or put it under tension, can also cause damage to the deeper cells in the hair follicle, and affect growth.

The principle behind the action of a hair conditioner

Hair conditioners are designed to prevent damage to the outer covering of the hair. The principles behind the actions of all types of hair conditioner are identical. The main functions of a hair conditioner are:

- to create a coating that covers the outer, rough layer of the hair – this coating gives the hair its smooth, uniform look;
- to neutralize the electric charges on the surface of the hair – by doing this, the hair does not look so 'wild' and unruly, and becomes much easier to comb and style; it also makes the hair look thicker and less wispy, and prevents 'knots'.

Note: The active ingredients in conditioners affect only the surface of the hair. They do not influence, nor do they not reach into the interior of the hair, and certainly they do not affect the hair follicle. Their effect is only temporary, and is lost within a few days (depending on environmental conditions), or if the hair is washed, then conditioners are removed from the surface of the hairs. The effect of a conditioner is purely cosmetic, and it does not have any medical benefits.

As with shampoos, apart from the active ingredient (which is the conditioner itself), these products also contain a variety of ingredients with various functions. They may contain fragrances, preservatives, moisturizers for dry hair, dyes, etc.

Types of hair conditioner

Hair conditioners can be of the following types:

- cationic surfactants
- cationic polymers
- protein conditioners

Cationic surfactants

In general, the surface of the damaged hair carries negative electric charges. Since cationic surfactants carry a positive electric charge, they are attracted to these negative charges and become attached to the surface of the hair.

Thus the outer surface of the hair acquires a uniform coating. At the same time the electric charges are neutralized.

Since cationic surfactants contain long fatty chains, they produce a fatty layer on the surface of the hair that gives it a soft, smooth feeling, and a shiny appearance.

Cationic surfactants are useful for hair that has been damaged as a result of dyeing, bleaching or waving. The more the outer surface of the hair is damaged, the more negative electric charges its surface carries, and the stronger the bond with the conditioner. The cationic surfactant is therefore attached most strongly to those areas of hair that are the most severely damaged, so the end result is that the surface of the hair develops a smooth, uniform look.

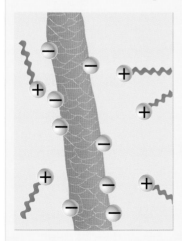

Mode of action of cationic surfactants.

Cationic polymers

In general, polymers are chemical compounds built up of long chains of many, small, identical building units. The cationic polymers that are used in hair conditioners contain substances such as:

- silicones,
- polyamides,
- polyamines,
- substances based on cellulose.

They become attached to the surface of the hair as long units of polymer chains.

Cationic polymers fill in the defects in the hair shaft, and thus allow light to be reflected more completely from the hair, since the hair surface is now smooth, continuous and uninterrupted.

These products are also cations (i.e. they carry a positive electric charge), so they also reduce the negative static electric charge on the surface of the hair. Shampoos containing cationic polymers are recommended for normal hair. Dermatologists do not recommend that they be used by those with delicate hair.

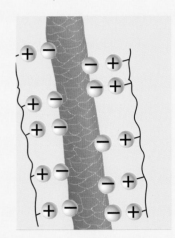

Mode of action of cationic polymers.

Protein conditioners

The protein in these conditioners is extracted from animal tissues (proteins such as keratin, collagen, casein and others), or from other sources, such as silk protein or plant proteins. The protein is made up of large molecules, and is therefore broken down into its components, which are of lower molecular weight (such as a mixture of peptides or amino acids). In that form (peptides or amino acids), they attach themselves to the hair and fill in the cracks and gaps. This strengthens the hair shaft, and repairs the split ends. It must be remembered that the hair shaft is not living tissue, so that it cannot bind the protein conditioners permanently. When the hair is washed, these substances are washed out of the hair shaft.

Protein conditioners penetrate into the cracks of the hair shaft.

How to use a hair conditioner

Hair conditioners are meant to be used after washing the hair with a shampoo. They should be applied **only to the hair**, and not the skin of the scalp. Most conditioners should be left on the hair for two to three minutes, and then rinsed off. For people with severely damaged hair, there are 'deep conditioners', which are left on the hair for several minutes (in accordance with the manufacturer's instructions) until being rinsed off.

Frequency of use of a hair conditioner

The frequency with which a hair conditioner is used varies in accordance with the need, and depends on the user's personal preference. People with healthy hair do not necessarily need a conditioner. If the hair has been damaged as a result of bleaching, waving or exposure to dry weather then a conditioner is helpful. If someone's hair tends to be unruly and 'all over the place', difficult to manage and to comb, and loses its lustre then a conditioner should be used.

Conditioners should not be used too much, since if an excessive amount settles on the hair, the hair tends to lose its 'live' look, and to become dull.

Hair styling: hair mousses and hair gels

Hair mousses and hair gels have a different task to that of a conditioner. **Mousses** are meant to help style the hair and help the hair keep its shape. They cover the hair with a thin, uniform coating that can protect the hair from unwanted external influences such as strong wind or strong sunlight. To create a specific hair style, **hair gels** are used. They make the hair firm, so that it can be styled into complex shapes, depending on the desired appearance.

28

Methods for temporary removal of hair

Contents Overview • Epilation and depilation: definitions • Methods of hair removal • Shaving • Mechanical scraping • Plucking • Chemical depilatories • Bleaching hair

Overview

People are becoming increasingly aware of the aesthetic aspects of their appearance. Men and women may be bothered by the presence of unwanted hair in certain areas. Most of the many methods currently available for hair removal provide only a temporary solution; other methods intended for the permanent removal of hair are discussed in Chapter 29. The present chapter reviews accepted methods for temporary removal of hair.

We must stress at this point several basic points:

- All people have hair follicles on most of the surface of their skin.
- The number of hair follicles in men and women is similar. The differences in the appearance of hair between men and women lie in the hair type: a hair follicle can produce a fine, thin, light (lacking pigment) hair that is almost invisible. This is called **vellus hair**. In contrast, other hair follicles may produce a long, thick, dark hair that is readily visible to the eye. That type of hair is called **terminal hair**. In children, the only terminal hair is on the scalp, the eyebrows, and the eyelashes. Facial hair in women and children is of the vellus hair type, which is not visible to the eye. The facial hair in men is of the terminal hair type, visible to the eye. Excessive hair in women refers to the fact that the thin, fine, almost invisible hair in various parts of the body becomes coarse, dark and visible.

Excessive hair: what causes it?

- **A high level of male hormones (e.g. testosterone) in the blood and body tissues:** Women normally have low basal levels of testosterone, but certain hormonal disturbances can occur, resulting in a rise in testosterone. In these cases, excessive hair will appear in places where hair typically is seen in males (such as facial hair). The appearance of excessive hair may be accompanied by other characteristics suggesting a hormonal basis for the problem, such as a deepening of the voice, irregularity of the menstrual cycle, persistent acne, an increase in muscle mass, and changes in the distribution of body fat.
- **Increased sensitivity of the hair follicles to normal hormone levels:** In this case, excessive hair appears, although the woman's basal level of testosterone will be within the normal limits. This phenomenon is attributed to increased sensitivity of the hair follicles to normal testosterone levels. The exact nature of this increased sensitivity is still unclear. The phenomenon is partly hereditary, and occurs more commonly in certain ethnic groups.

In every case of excessive hair in a woman, it is not sufficient to merely remove the excess hair cosmetically – the woman should also be referred for a medical endocrinological (hormonal) evaluation, which will include examination by a gynaecologist and/or an endocrinologist.

However, there are many women who need or desire to remove hair from various parts of the body even without having any medical problem. This chapter discusses the accepted methods for the removal of hair.

Epilation and depilation: definitions

Epilation
Epilation is a technique whereby the hair is removed by its root. However, not all epilation techniques will also destroy the active cells at the hair root. Depending on the particular type of epilation method, the hair may be eliminated temporarily or permanently. Electrolysis, for example, is a method of epilation that aims to eliminate hair permanently (see Chapter 29). On the other hand, plucking the hair (using wax or a thread), is a method of epilation where the hair is only removed temporarily.

Depilation
Depilation is a method of hair removal that does not involve the root of the hair, but a region higher up the hair shaft, at or near the surface of the skin. Examples of depilation are shaving and the use of depilatory creams. All depilation methods only remove hair temporarily.

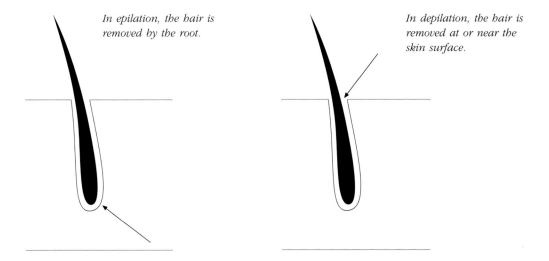

In epilation, the hair is removed by the root.

In depilation, the hair is removed at or near the skin surface.

Methods of hair removal

These include:

- shaving
- mechanical scraping
- various methods of plucking (tweezers, thread, warm wax, melted sugar, cold wax, or special instruments)
- chemical depilatories

Shaving

Shaving is fast, simple, convenient and painless. Many women use this method for shaving their legs and armpits. It can be used on the face, but women, in general, prefer not to shave the face because of the masculine connotation of that procedure.

Note: The myth that shaving the hair increases the rate of growth and produces thicker hair is without foundation. The upper part of the hair that is found above the surface of the skin does not contain any living material. This upper part is composed of lifeless keratinous tissue, and therefore cutting or shaving it cannot result in the growth of coarse, thick, dark hair, and does not encourage hair growth. When a hair (which, as stated, is merely dead keratinous material) is cut, there is no effect on the hair root where the active cells that cause the hair grow are found. The mistaken impression arose, perhaps, because the short hairs (stubble) that are seen on the skin after hair is shaved are straight, prickly, and relatively thick compared with their length, with a severed end. As the hair grows longer, it loses its 'prickliness'.

Advantages of shaving

Shaving is not painful, it is quick and safe, it can be used over wide areas of skin, and it can be used on any type of skin and any hair – fair or dark.

Disadvantages of shaving

- The main disadvantage is that the hair grows back relatively soon after its shaving and has to be reshaved.
- Skin may be nicked.
- There may be skin irritation.
- Bacterial infection in the shaved area may occur. These infections (medically termed as **folliculitis**) tend to occur more frequently in the groin.

To prevent cuts, skin irritation and infections, it is advisable:

- to use a new, sharp blade;
- to soften the skin by wetting the area to be shaved and covering it with a sufficient layer of lather;
- to shave as gently as possible, with minimal pressure of the blade on the skin.

In cases where the skin tends to be injured, each stroke of the blade should be directed towards a new area of hair, and a stroke of only a few millimetres should be used each time – this is preferable to trying to cover wide areas of skin in one movement. In this situation, once the hair has been 'soaked' in water and lather, the excess lather should be removed so that the precise location of the short hairs, and their direction of growth, can be seen in order that they can be shaved correctly.

Mechanical scraping

Another method, equivalent to shaving, is mechanical scraping. In its classic form this is done using a **pumice stone**. As with shaving, this procedure needs to be repeated every few days. Vigorous scraping, which may result in redness and irritation of the skin, should be avoided. A similar technique is to rub the skin gently in a circular motion with a **depilatory glove**, whose surface is composed of fine sandpaper.

An antiseptic alcohol solution should be applied before scraping the skin. Following the scraping, moisturizers containing 'soothing' preparations (such as aloe vera or witch hazel) should be applied.

Plucking

In shaving, the hair is cut off at the skin surface, at the level of the dead keratinous component of the hair; therefore there is no effect on processes that occur in the live region of the hair root. On the other hand, by plucking, the

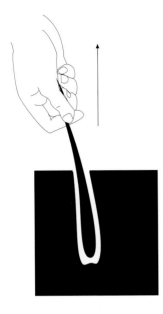

Pulling a hair out by the roots by plucking.

hair root is **actively pulled out**, and the consequences are unpredictable and change from person to person.

Repeated plucking can cause some damage to the hair root. In most cases, plucking has no effect on the shape or structure of the hair (for example, many women pluck their eyebrows without this causing coarse, dark, thick hair to grow back). However, the reaction of the eyebrow's hair to its plucking is unpredictable, differing from one person to another. Sometimes plucked hair follicles of the eyebrows tend to grow hairs that turn in different directions, deviating from the natural direction of the eyebrow hair. On the other hand, and relatively more commonly, following repeated plucking, the hair tends to become finer and thinner. Note that in the area of the eyebrows, after plucking (or repeated plucking), the hair may not grow back. Often the recovery period following the plucking of eyebrow hair is relatively long, and may last for more than one year. Therefore unnecessary plucking in this area should be avoided. Many women who 'succumbed' to fashion trends of the past are now forced to draw-in their eyebrows because the eyebrow hair has thinned out owing to repeated plucking.

Does the hair become thicker and coarser after plucking?

Sometimes there is the impression that, following plucking, the hair becomes thicker and coarser. In most cases, that appearance is not a result of the plucking, but rather a reflection of the normal life cycle of the hair: a hair follicle that is plucked while it is in the resting (telogen) phase, will later be in the active (anagen) phase, with new hair growing from it. The new hair grows, and because it is in the active anagen phase, it can look thick, dark and coarse. However, this is merely a reflection of the particular phase of the hair's life cycle at that time, and is not related to the plucking.

Different methods of plucking include:

- tweezers
- thread
- warm or cold wax; warm melted sugar
- special instruments

Possible disadvantage of plucking
- There may be pain – which some people cannot tolerate.
- Folliculitis (inflammation of the hair follicles) may occur. This is caused by microscopic injuries during plucking, and subsequent infection by bacteria.
- Scars may develop in the areas of plucked hair.

Main advantage of plucking
As opposed to shaving, the smooth, hairless skin left behind after plucking remains that way for a longer time. The hair tends not to grow back for a few weeks in areas that have been plucked.

Using tweezers or a thread
Plucking with tweezers or a thread is used where there are a small number of hairs to be removed (such as the eyebrows, chin, etc.), or where there are isolated hairs in some part of the body (for example around the nipples). The thread is coiled around the hair and allows it to be plucked out easily and efficiently.

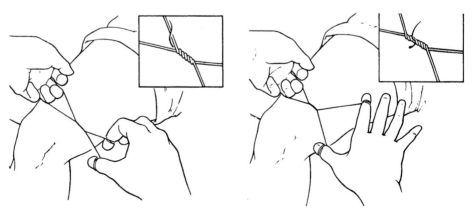

Plucking a hair using a thread.

Warm wax
Using wax to remove hair is, in fact, a form of plucking that can be done over relatively wide areas of skin. The wax that is used is obtained from beehives.

The treatment is performed as follows: The wax is heated until it melts, and is smeared over the area where the hairs are about to be removed. The wax solidifies within a minute, and the hairs become stuck to the wax and 'trapped' in it. The layer of solid wax can then be peeled away rapidly from the skin, pulling away the hair 'trapped' within it. Using wax detaches hairs from the skin near the root – deeper than the effect of shaving, which removes the hair at the skin surface – so the effect lasts longer than the effect of shaving. It takes a few weeks for plucked hairs to reappear above the surface of the skin.

A few days after using wax, new hairs may appear. This is not regrowth of the plucked hairs, but growth of new hair that happened to be in the active growth phase of its life cycle. These hairs were due to appear in that area regardless of the wax treatment.

Using warm wax: instructions before applying the wax

- Thoroughly clean and dry the skin.
- Some people recommend sprinkling a light layer of talc on the skin to absorb any residual moisture or oil, so the wax will stick better to the skin.
- When using warm wax, make sure that it is not too hot by testing a drop on the back of the hand.
- Never use wax on injured or diseased skin.
- There is no point in advising wax treatment for someone who has recently shaved the area or used a chemical depilatory agent, since the hair in the area will be too short and will not become stuck in the wax. In such a case, wait two or three weeks until the hair has grown longer.

Applying the wax

- Smear the wax on the skin in the direction of the hair growth.
- Wait a few minutes for it to cool and harden, and remove it (with the attached hairs) by peeling if off against the direction of the hair growth.

Following the treatment

- Disinfect the skin with alcohol.

Disadvantages of warm wax

- Wax is only partly effective, since it cannot 'trap' and hence cannot remove short hairs that have just reached the surface of the skin; hairs of less than 2 mm in length are usually not caught up in the wax.
- Irritant or allergic reactions may occur – ranging from mild irritation (manifested by transient redness and slight stinging) to moderate and severe reactions. If there is merely a mild skin irritation, it is sufficient to apply soothing preparations (such as 1% hydrocortisone cream or aloe vera preparations) on the affected skin. In the case of more severe reactions, the patient should be referred to a dermatologist.

- Folliculitis (inflammation of the hair follicles) may appear following waxing. It is manifested by the appearance of many small, red lesions, or by the presence of many small lesions containing pus, where the hairs grow. In this case, the patient must be referred to a dermatologist.
- The technique may be painful; different people feel the pain to different degrees.
- Burns: careless use of hot wax may burn the skin.
- Waxing may cause the appearance of superficial small blood vessels on the skin.

In most women who have used wax for years, specific or significant problems do not occur. There have been reports that, after prolonged use of wax, there is less regrowth of hair, and the hair that does regrow tends to be finer and thinner. Theoretically, that is possible, because repeatedly plucking out of a hair by the root does damage the root. Nevertheless, most women who use wax find that they have to continue treatment time after time, for years, so that the above effect, if it does occur, is insignificant.

Warm melted sugar

This is not popular, because it is painful. The technique is based on applying warm, melted sugar, which is sticky, then pulling it off together with the hairs that have stuck to it. A strip of material is used to help pull out those hairs that have stuck to the sugar. The method is similar to warm wax treatment.

Cold wax

Cold wax works the same way as does warm wax – the hair is 'trapped' in the cold wax, which is then quickly peeled off, thus plucking out the trapped hair. To be precise, the correct chemical term for 'cold wax' is, in fact, not wax at all, but a mixture of various sugars. Usually these preparations also contain citric acid. This combination of compounds produces a thick and sticky substance, which is generally quite effective in pulling out hairs. In general, the stickier the substance, the easier it is to remove the hair, and the less painful it is.

Special instruments for plucking

The various instruments on the market for plucking hair are based on the action of a spiral spring. The hair is caught up in the spring and pulled out. The pros and cons of this technique are the same as those of plucking hair in general, but the design of these instruments allows hair to be removed quickly from the limbs.

Chemical depilatories

These preparations are marketed as creams or ointments; some are also available as gels or foams or in a roll-on form.

Chemical depilatories contain chemical substances that dissolve the keratin fibres from which the external part of the hair is made. The hair comes off at or just below skin level, The hairs tend to break in those places where the keratin is slightly deficient or unevenly distributed.

Chemical depilatories affect only the external part of the hair, and not the living root. Therefore, within a few days, the hairs growing back can be noticed.

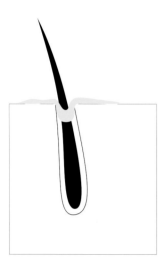

Hair comes away at the skin surface when it is treated with depilatory cream.

Main types of preparations

Sulfides
Barium sulfide and strontium sulfide have been used since 1800; they act rapidly and effectively. However, when using these substances, a compound called hydrogen sulfide (H_2S) is formed, which has a repellent 'rotten egg' smell and irritates the skin.

Thioglycolates
These form the main component of the preparations that are currently used. The basic ingredient of depilatory agents is a salt of thioglycolic acid. These compounds act on the fibres of the hair, dissolving and disrupting the keratin.

Thioglycolate salts tend to cause less skin irritation than do the sulfides, and their odour is also less of a problem; however, it takes longer for the hair to come away from the skin. Because thioglycolates rarely cause skin irritation, they are designed for use on areas of sensitive skin, such as the face. The length of application time is determined by the manufacturer, and is usually between 5 and 20 minutes, depending on the nature of the preparation and the strength of the hair. These preparations work well on fine hair.

Enzymatic depilatory agents

There is no problem of odour or skin irritation with these substances. The basic component is an enzyme called **keratinase**, which dissolves the protein of the keratin that makes up the hair. The enzyme is produced by certain bacteria. These compounds are less effective than the two groups of substances discussed above.

Instructions for use of depilatory agents

- Follow the manufacturer's directions carefully; the instructions may vary depending on the type and concentration of the preparation.
- Do not leave the preparation on the skin for longer than is specified in the instructions.
- Do not apply to the face a cream meant for the legs.
- Do not use these creams on damaged skin; in any case of skin disease, a dermatologist should be consulted.
- The first time a preparation is used, it should be tried on a small area of skin (usually the arm) first to confirm that there is no abnormal sensitivity to the substance. Evaluation of the test area should be done after 24–48 hours.If after that trial application there is no skin irritation (redness, swelling, itching or burning sensation), the substance can be used over wider areas of skin.
- Clean and dry the skin thoroughly before using the depilatory agent.
- The skin adjacent to the area to be treated can be protected by covering it with a fatty preparation, such as petroleum jelly.
- After leaving the depilatory agent on for the required time, wash it off with lukewarm water.

Advantage of depilatory agents

The main advantage, compared with other methods is that they are painless.

Disadvantages of depilatory agents

- There may be skin irritation – chemical depilatories may affect not only the hairs, but also the superficial layers of the skin. This irritation is due to the fact that both the hair and the skin are composed of keratin. The degree and extent of irritation depend on the type of preparation (more common with the sulfides) and its concentration. Mild irritation may be treated by application of 1% hydrocortisone cream or aloe vera preparations. In more severe cases, the patient should be referred to a physician.
- They can give rise to an unpleasant odour.
- Regrowth of the hair can occur following the use of a depilatory agent. Although the hair is removed at a deeper level than with shaving, within a few days, the hairs growing back can be noticed.

Bleaching hair

This is another method of dealing with the problem of excess hair. It is intended for women with a fair complexion who wish to 'camouflage' hair on the face and arms. The hair is still there, but is less obvious and almost invisible.

A bleaching preparation can be made by mixing hydrogen peroxide with ammonia, in a low concentration. The effect of the solution starts immediately after the two substances are mixed. There are many preparations on the market for bleaching hair. The preparation should be applied, and left on the area to be treated for 5–15 minutes, depending on the manufacturer's instructions.

Note: As is usual with cosmetic agents, the first time a bleaching preparation is used, it is advisable to try it out on a small, unexposed area of skin. Only when it has been confirmed that the substance is safe should it be used over a wider area.

If there is a burning sensation, the bleach should be washed off with water. The application can be tried again a few days later with a weaker solution – once the burning sensation has disappeared completely.

If the treatment was not adequate to achieve the desired result, it can be repeated a day or two later, with the bleach being left on the skin a little longer this time.

29

Permanent hair removal: Electrolysis–electric needle

Contents Permanent removal of hair • Electrolysis: overview • Equipment needed for electrolysis • Instructions for electrolysis • When should electrolysis not be performed • Complications of electrolysis • Effectiveness of electrolysis

Note: To better understand the boxed sections in this chapter, the reader should review Chapter 25 on the structure of hair, particularly the section dealing with the growth cycle of hair.

Permanent removal of hair

Electrolysis has been proven to be effective in permanently removing hair. Another technique for dealing with excess hair is by the use of a laser. Laser treatment stops the active growth period of the hair for long periods. The use of lasers for removing hair is discussed in Chapter 23. Apart from these two methods, there are other techniques on the market that claim to remove hair permanently. Some are based on a series of treatments with gel preparations that contain various substances (some contain aromatic oils) combined with equipment for heating the gel, and the hair is then removed with wax.

Note: Apart from laser treatment and electrolysis, the results of no other techniques for the permanent removal of hair have been published or proved in the accepted scientific literature. Hence we have no objective way of assessing whether those methods are effective.

The term 'permanent removal of hair' applies only to the treated hair follicles – and even then the results are not absolute (see the final section of this chapter, on the effectiveness of electrolysis). In the skin area treated by electrolysis, there may be hair follicles that were not treated by the electric needle (i.e. follicles that were not in the stage of active growth) or hair follicles that were ineffectively treated. However, when speaking about a single hair follicle that has been effectively treated, irreversible damage is expected to have occurred, and this follicle will not grow a new hair.

Electrolysis: overview

Electrolysis is an effective method for the permanent removal of hair, based on inserting a fine metal needle into the hair follicle, with the aim of destroying the active cells in the hair root. At this point, let us recall that a **hair follicle** is an elongated tube-like depression, in which a hair grows. At the base of the follicle are the active cells of the hair root, responsible for its growth. Hence, to destroy these active cells, a fine metal needle is inserted through the opening of the follicle at the skin, and advanced until the tip reaches the base of the follicle. At this stage, an electric current is passed down the needle to destroy the active cells at the hair root. The hair breaks off at the root, and can then be easily pulled with fine tweezers.

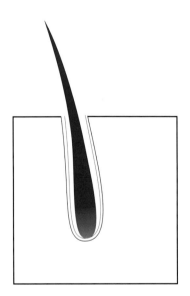

Hair follicle (shown in red).

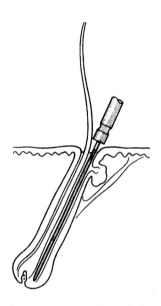

Insertion of a needle to the base of the hair root.

The great advantage of this technique derives from the fact that a follicle that has been effectively treated by the electric needle cannot grow a hair again – provided that the active cells in the root have indeed been destroyed.

Note: The illustrations on pages 294, 297, 298 and 299 are presented by courtesy of Dr RN Richards, from the book *Cosmetic and Medical Electrolysis and Temporary Hair Removal*, by RN Richards and GE Meharg (Medric Ltd, Second edn, 1997). This book is recommended for those who are interested in additional information on electrolysis.

Equipment needed for electrolysis

Several types of electrolysis equipment are in use in cosmetic clinics. We shall discuss the general features of each one:

1 direct electrolysis
2 electrocoagulation
3 blend
4 instruments for home use

1 Direct electrolysis

This method, less commonly used nowadays, is based on the use of a direct electric current (galvanic current) that destroys the cells in the hair follicle. The main disadvantages of this method are:

- the need for a prolonged electric current of a minute or more for each hair
- pain

The main advantage of the method is that it is much more effective than other electrolysis techniques.

Direct electrolysis

The remarkable effectiveness of this technique stems from the mode of action on the hair cells. The electric current results in the production of a chemical substance – **sodium hydroxide (NaOH)** – that destroys the cells of the hair root. The sodium hydroxide trickles down the length of the follicle, reaches the cells at the root, and destroys them.

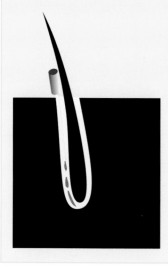

Production of sodium hydroxide, which moves down to the active cells at the hair root and destroys them.

2 Electrocoagulation

This is a newer technique, which is now commonly used in cosmetic clinics. It uses a high-frequency electric current to destroy the hair root by creating heat in the follicle. Other names for this method include:

- diathermy
- thermolysis
- high-frequency alternating method
- short-wave

Electrocoagulation involves the use of a high-frequency alternating current. The current passes along the needle and heats up the tissues of the hair follicle, destroying them. With this instrument, the current is applied for only a few seconds.

Another technique, known as **high-speed flash thermolysis**, involves applying the current for less than a second. The significant advantage of this technique compared with ordinary electrocoagulation is its speed. Using this procedure, it is possible to remove up to 200 hairs in an hour. However, it causes less destruction to the tissues at the base of the hair, and is less effective in removing coarse hairs.

3 Blend

This method combines direct electrolysis and electrocoagulation, and is more effective for the removal of coarse hairs.

4 Instruments for home use

The principle of use of these instruments is similar to the techniques described above, but the electric current is provided by batteries. The needle is inserted into the hair follicle until the end of the needle reaches the hair root, the electric current is then applied to destroy the root.

The main disadvantages of home use are that, since the user is not a professional, it is difficult to treat certain areas, such as the face; the user must get accustomed to working with a mirror; and treating oneself tends to be slow. In general, this method is not recommended for areas with extensive hair.

Needles

- Use only disposable needles.
- The length and diameter of the needle should be appropriate for the type of hair being removed. If the needle is too thick, it cannot be inserted into the hair follicle. On the other hand, if the needle is too small, the treatment will be less painful – but also less effective.

- The upper part of the needle should be covered by insulating material, to prevent damage and scarring to the upper layers of the skin.
- A relatively flexible needle, made of two parts, is preferable to a rigid needle. This enables it to be inserted into the hair follicle more precisely.

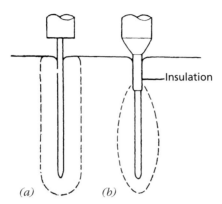

(a) An epilation needle. (b) A needle with insulating material at its upper end: this insulation prevents unnecessary damage to the upper part of the hair follicle (there is no point in destroying this part, anyhow), and to the skin surface. The cells one wants to destroy are in the hair root, at the base of the follicle.

Instructions for electrolysis

1 In order to enable the operator to achieve the high level of concentration needed, the client should be lying down, while the operator is seated nearby, as comfortably as possible.
2 Bright light and a magnifying glass are essential for an effective treatment.
3 The region to be treated should be shaved three to five days before the treatment.
4 Apply antiseptic solution (e.g. chlorhexidine, alcoholic solutions) before and after the treatment. Following electrolysis, some cosmeticians apply a substance with a cooling and soothing effect, such as witch hazel. Some recommend the application of 0.5–1% hydrocortisone cream, which has anti-inflammatory properties.
5 During the procedure itself:
   - Insert the needle into the opening of the follicle and advance it gently and precisely as much as possible within the follicle. A sensation of touching a 'barrier' is felt when the needle has reached the base of the follicle.
   - Use the correct current strength, in accordance with the manufacturer's instructions. In the newer instruments, in common use these days, the duration of the current is controlled automatically.

Why shave the region to be treated?

The reason for shaving the area to be treated is so that one can identify those hairs that are in the **anagen** phase. Those are the hairs that grow back after shaving. As opposed to the scalp, where 60% of the hairs are in anagen, only 30–50% of body hairs are in the anagen phase. Identifying those hairs that are in the anagen phase allows the treatment to be carried out on those hairs; electrolysis carried out on anagen hairs is very effective, whereas if it is carried out on hairs in the telogen phase it is much less effective.

The reason why electrolysis on hairs in the telogen phase is less effective is that, in that situation, the base of the follicle where the needle tip reaches is actually the root of the old hair; when a hair is in the telogen phase, it is almost impossible to reach the place from which the new hair will start growing.

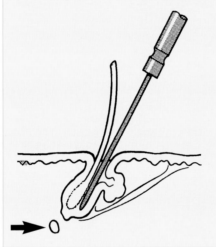

Ineffectual insertion of the needle into a follicle that is in the telogen phase. The new hair will grow from the part of the follicle indicated by the arrow: the needle cannot get to that place while the hair is in the telogen phase.

Minimizing the pain associated with electrolysis

The degree of pain experienced during electrolysis varies, depending on the pain threshold of the individual patient, and on the region of the body being treated.

Consider using **EMLA cream** for patients who have a low pain threshold or for treatment of particularly sensitive areas, such as the upper lip, the groins, and around the nipples. EMLA cream (Eutectic Mixture of Lidocaine and Prilocaine) contains local anaesthetic agents – a mixture of lidocaine and prilocaine. The cream is applied to the skin about 60 minutes before the treatment, and an occlusive dressing applied over it. EMLA may reduce the pain considerably. While using EMLA, one should be cautious: minimizing the pain means also losing an important parameter of the degree of possible damage to the skin.

During electrolysis, try to avoid the following pitfalls:

1 **Avoid activating the electric current while the needle is located superficially in the follicle.** If the needle is too superficial (not deep enough) and does not reach the hair root, the electric current will not destroy the active cells that form the hair. Furthermore, there is a risk of damage to the skin, resulting in scarring.

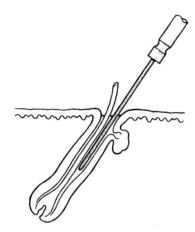

Too-superficial placement of the needle.

2 **Avoid puncturing the follicle wall.** If the needle passes through the wall of the follicle, into the surrounding tissue, there will be damage to the skin tissue, and hair growth will not be affected. This tends to occur in a 'crooked' hair follicle, in which case the operator will find it hard to insert the needle correctly. A deviation of one or two millimetres from the correct direction of the electrolysis needle may result in damage to the follicle wall or to the skin near the follicle.

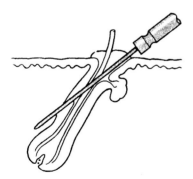

Needle passing through the wall of the follicle, and 'missing' the active cells in the hair root.

3 **When electrolysis is performed in the armpits and groin, take extreme care.** In these areas, certain anatomical structures (e.g. nerves and lymph nodes) are located near to the surface of the skin. It is advisable to fold the skin between two fingers in order to elevate the area being treated from the skin surface and to prevent possible damage to these structures.

When should electrolysis not be performed?

1 Do not carry out electrolysis on injured skin, or skin affected by any disease.
2 If the client suffers from any disease (e.g. heart disease, especially those with a car-diac pacemaker), obtain a doctor's written permission before using electrolysis.
3 Clients suffering from an infectious disease (e.g. AIDS or viral hepatitis) can undergo electrolysis, but extra care must be taken:
   • **take extreme care not to get jabbed by the needle;**
   • **in any case, use only disposable needles for every patient.**
4 Electrolysis should not be used to remove hairs growing from naevi. The cells that make up a naevus are **melanocytes**, which are the cells that produce the pigment melanin. Some of the destructive skin tumours, such as melanomas, arise from melanocytes. One cannot predict the possible influence of an elec-tric current on these cells, and hence it should be avoided. In such cases, the patient should be referred to a dermatologist or a plastic surgeon, who will remove the naevus in its entirety.
5 Do not carry out electrolysis on hair that is next to cartilage (e.g. the ear or nose).
6 Check with the patient whether he/she has a tendency to form raised scars, or dark hyperpigmented scars (ask about previous operations or injuries, and what the scars look like). If there is a possibility of these problems, treat a few hairs in an area that is not readily visible, wait a few months, and then evaluate the out-come. In someone who tends to produce raised scars after the slightest injury, a dermatologist's opinion should be sought before embarking on electrolysis.
7 In women with excessive hair (**hirsutism**) there may be a hormonal problem, which could have significant medical implications. In such cases, a medical opinion must be obtained to determine whether, in fact, such a problem exists. Should that be the case, the physician may consider hormonal treatment together with, or prior to, the electrolysis treatment.

Complications of electrolysis

In general, most of the complications from electrolysis arise from damage to the skin while carrying out the procedure. That is not surprising, since the damage results from the very mechanism that is used to destroy the hair root. **The aim of treatment is that the damage (deliberately) caused by the electroly-sis should be confined to the hair root alone.** However, it is obvious that incorrect placement of the needle, or using a current that is higher than neces-sary, will cause damage to the tissues around the follicle. This damage will be manifested as follows:

1 An **inflammatory reaction**, such as reddening and mild swelling in the area of the follicle, may appear.
2 There may be **scarring.** Used correctly, it is rare for electrolysis to result in scarring. If there is mild, superficial damage to the opening of the hair follicle, small scabs may appear over the openings of the treated hair follicles. These

scabs usually disappear within a few days. However, should there be a more severe reaction, permanent scars may result. Scars may result from:

- inserting the needle too superficially – the electric current then passes next to the surface of the skin;
- using too strong an electric current;
- not applying the current at all, or not applying it to the base of the hair – the scar appears following the hair being pulled out;
- infection.

In certain people, usually those with dark skin, there may be a tendency to produce excessive scarring following injuries, operations etc. These scars are dark in colour and raised. Particular care must be taken when treating these people. If it is suspected that the patient does have that problem (either from the patient's history or by examining his/her skin) then electrolysis should be avoided. A test can be performed by treating a few hair follicles in an area that is not readily visible, and waiting to see the outcome. In any case, it is advisable to consult a dermatologist before deciding upon electrolysis treatment in such patients.

Other possible complications

These include the following:

- Infection may develop in the treated area – either because of lack of adequate sterile technique or because of widespread tissue damage. In that case, a physician will need to prescribe antibiotics, which may involve only the external application of an antibiotic cream or ointment. However, in more serious or widespread infections the patient may need to take antibiotic capsules or tablets.
- Infection may be spread from one patient to another – hence the importance of using disposable needles.
- A rare occurrence is for a needle to break inside the skin. This uncommon event does not usually pose a serious problem, and the broken-off needle can usually be removed from the skin without too much difficulty. If the point of the needle is in the skin and cannot be removed, a doctor will have to deal with it.

Effectiveness of electrolysis

Since electrolysis is mainly performed by cosmeticians, rather than doctors, the results of treatment are not subject to statistical analysis. There is relatively little information on this subject in the medical literature. Furthermore, the outcome will vary from operator to operator, since it depends very much on his/her skill and experience.

In general, the process is slow, exhausting and expensive, since the needle has to be inserted separately into each hair follicle. The advantage of electrolysis, however, is that if it is performed correctly and effectively, it destroys the hair follicle permanently.

Most clients can have between 50 and 100 follicles dealt with at one treatment session. Accordingly, several months of treatment are needed to remove all the hair from a relatively small area of skin, such as the upper lip or the chin. In cases of marked hirsutism, it may take two or three years of weekly treatments to achieve the desired result.

Has the hair root been permanently destroyed?

Since the hair is pulled out and removed during the treatment in any case (whether the electric current was on or not), a certain period must elapse before one can ascertain whether the hair root was destroyed for good.

- If the hair was in the telogen phase, it will grow back a few weeks later.
- If the hair was in the anagen phase, several months will have to elapse before one can be certain whether the hair root was destroyed permanently or not.

Reappearance of hair

Hair that reappears in an area that was treated by electrolysis can be the result of the following:

- Hair follicles that were not treated correctly.
- If hair appears relatively quickly (within a few days of treatment), it is reasonable to assume that those hairs were in the early growth phase (early anagen), and were not visible above the surface at the time of the electrolysis, so those follicles were, in fact not treated at all.
- If the hair in the treated area appears some time later, it is possible that those hairs were in the telogen phase at the time of treatment, and were not treated, or that the treatment was not effective and they are now in the anagen phase.
- Another possibility is that the fine, vellus hair is slowly changing to coarser hair. This occurs more frequently in women with a hormonal problem, and in such cases the underlying medical problem should be diagnosed. The only way to prevent endless cosmetic treatments is to treat the basic hormonal problem, since there is no point in treating hair with an electric needle if, all the while, there is a constant stimulus acting that keeps making the hair darker, coarser and more obvious.

Various estimates suggest that about 30–40% of the hair will reappear following electrolysis. Direct electrolysis, using a direct (galvanic) current, is much more effective. However, some dermatologists do not agree with these results, and maintain that the outcome of electrolysis treatment is not nearly as good as that.

30
The nails

Contents Overview • Composition of the nails • Structure of the nails • General care of the nails • Common nail problems • Cosmetic treatment of nails • Artificial nails

Overview

Human nails are the equivalent to the claws in other mammals; however the functions of the nails as tools or weapons have, with evolution, become less important. Nowadays, the function of the nails in humans is basically to protect the fingers and to assist in delicate manual activities.

The presence of healthy nails, of aesthetically pleasing appearance, is very significant. Nails that are well cared for complement a pleasant overall appearance, and also reflect one's general health status. To some extent, the nails may also reflect a person's social status.

Composition of the nails

The nails are made up largely of **keratin** – the same protein that makes up the hair and the skin – although here we are talking of a special variant of keratin. Nails are composed of '**hard keratin**', which is similar in its chemical composition to the substance that animals' horns are made of. This form of keratin contains much more sulfur than the normal skin keratin. In addition, nails contain small amounts of elements such as calcium, iron and zinc.

The relative flexibility of nails is due to the presence of compounds called **phospholipids**. These are fatty compounds that also contain polysaccharides and proteins. Phospholipids are the major component of cell membranes in the body.

Water can pass through the nails readily – more so than through the skin – so that repeated contact with water and cleansing agents causes the nails to become relatively dry, and more brittle.

The strength of the nails is not only related to their composition, but also to their shape. The convex shape of a normal nail makes it stronger than it would be if it were flat.

Structure of the nails

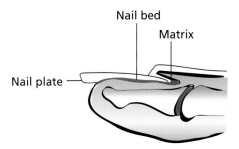

Structure of the nail.

Nail plate
This is the external, visible part of the nail.

Nail matrix
The definition of the term 'matrix', in its broad sense, is 'environment or tissue that gives origin or form to something'. The term 'nail matrix' refers, therefore, to the root of the nail. This is the living, active part of the nail. The cells of the nail matrix are in the area of the **lunula** (see below) and under the skin fold at the nail base. Matrix cells are continuously dividing, and thus the nail grows.

Any injury or damage to the nail matrix may distort the nail. Severe, permanent damage to the nail matrix will result in permanent deformity of the nail, even to the extent of its total loss.

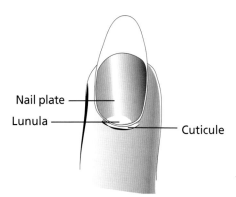

The lunula and cuticle of the nail.

Lunula
The lunula is the pale, crescent-like structure found at the base of the nail. It represents the visible front part of the nail matrix from which the nail grows.

Similarities between hair growth and nail growth

In the same way that, in hair, the cells at the base that are dividing continuously result in the hair growing (the external hair being dead keratinous material), in a nail the cells at the base divide and the nail grows longer. The outer part of the nail is also composed of dead keratinous (horny) material.

Differences between hair growth and nail growth

In the nail, as stated earlier, the keratin that is formed is of a different type to that of the hair. And, in contrast to hair, which has growth cycles, nails grow continuously and steadily throughout life.

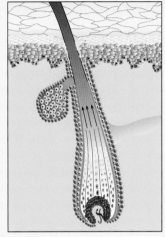

Hair growth

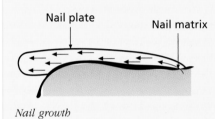

Nail growth

Nail bed

The nail bed is the soft tissue underneath the nail plate. It contains many tiny blood vessels, which give the nail its pink colour. The actual nail plate itself (as can be seen at the edge of the nail that protrudes beyond the edge of the finger) is white.

Cuticle

This is the skin fold at the base of the nail.

Some data regarding nail growth

Fingernails grow approximately 3–4 mm per month; toenails grow more slowly, approximately at 40% of the growth rate of fingernails. Nail growth is influenced by the weather: it is accelerated in warm weather and becomes slower in cold temperatures.

Growth is influenced by age: nails grow faster in younger people. Advanced age is accompanied by a gradual slowing down of the nail growth rate.

Using the fingers (e.g. typing) stimulates nail growth, so that in right-handed people the fingernails on the right hand grow a little faster than those of the left hand.

Some medications may alter the rate of nail growth. Nails grow faster during pregnancy.

General care of the nails

Nail care

- Nails should not be regarded as instruments (e.g. for opening lids, tabs of drink cans, etc.). Long nails that protrude beyond the edges of the fingers tend to break more readily, so that it may not be a good idea to grow long nails.
- Nail biting should be avoided.
- Repeated exposure to water eventually leads to drying out and damage to the nails. The nails become more brittle, and tend to split at their ends. Also, exposing the nails to soap and cleansing agents leads to dryness and damage.

Therefore, when washing dishes or performing some activity involving exposure to various chemicals, it is advisable to wear protective gloves, (as explained in detail in Chapter 13 on inflammation and dermatitis), particularly if there is frequent exposure to water or chemicals.

Cutting the nails

The hands should be rinsed in warm water prior to cutting the nails in order to soften the nails. While cutting, the nail should be rounded at its front edge; however, its sides should be left straight.

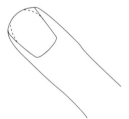
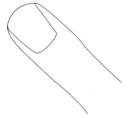

Improper cutting of the nail (indicated by the dashes), with an attempt at rounding off the nail's natural, straight line.   *The proper way of cutting the nail.*

Unnecessary rounding off of the corners of the nail should be avoided. The nail should not be cut beyond its natural line of growth. If care is taken to cut the nails this way, they will be stronger. Furthermore, this prevents the occurrence of an **ingrown nail** ('hangnail') which is the painful penetration of the nail into the surrounding tissues.

Common nail problems

Nail deformities

Deformation, or a change in nail shape, may indicate a medical problem, which in some cases may be diagnosed merely from the shape of the nail. Covering or hiding the misshapen nail(s) with artificial nails may interfere with the correct diagnosis of the problem by a physician – thus further damage may occur, leading to permanent nail deformity.

Therefore, it is advisable to seek medical advice from a dermatologist if there is nail deformity. Only after the medical evaluation has been completed may artificial nails be used.

In many cases, nail deformity is the result of fungal infection. In recent years, many effective medications against fungal infections of the nails have been developed, so in most cases these infections can now be cured.

Note: The earlier the patient sees the doctor, the better are the chances of full recovery. The longer a nail deformity has been present, if it involves the nail matrix, the less are the chances of complete recovery.

Brittle nails

As mentioned above, changes in the shape of the nail may reflect some medical problem (skin disease or internal disease). Nevertheless, not every change in the nail necessarily means that there is an underlying medical problem.

Brittleness and splitting of the nails are common, and occur more often in women than in men. Although it is true that excessive brittleness of the nails may be due to a general illness (including malnutrition and anorexia), the commonest cause is dryness of the nails as a result of repeated exposure to water and cleansing agents. Even simple washing of the hands, if carried out too frequently, can cause brittleness of the nails. Excessive exposure to cleansing agents (such as dishwashing liquid), or over-frequent use of nail polish removers, damage the keratin, the water content of the nails decreases, and they become more brittle.

The main principles of treatment of brittle nails include:

- prevention of exposure of the nails to repeated wetting, cleansing agents and other chemicals – protective gloves should be used (use cotton gloves, with seams outside, beneath plastic gloves: see p. 141);
- phospholipid-containing cream should be applied to the nail after each hand wash (see below).

In addition, there are those who recommend taking various vitamins or other basic elements (mainly metals) as treatment for brittle nails (biotin and zinc are commonly recommended). A physician may consider the use of substances such as these in certain cases of brittle nails.

Cosmetic treatment of nails

General: manicure

The term **manicure** describes the variety of treatments related to care of the fingernails. The word is derived from the Latin *manus* = hand, *cura* = care (similar to the term **pedicure** – care of the foot and the toenails: *pedis* = foot). Manicure includes the following:

Cutting the nails correctly
As discussed above, the nail should be rounded at its front edge; the corners should not be rounded off, but left squared. Cutting the nails correctly helps to strengthen them, and prevents the development of ingrown nails (hangnail).

Smoothing the free edge of the nail
This is done using a nail file or an emery board.

Care of the cuticle
The cuticle is the skin fold at the base of the nail. The management of the cuticle basically consists of cutting away excess skin in such a way as to make this part of the nail look neater (if necessary). This is done after gently freeing the cuticle from the nail plate. Before trimming the cuticles, soaking the fingers in warm water for several minutes to soften the skin is recommended. It is advisable to use special cuticle-softening oils.

To free the cuticle from the nail plate and to trim it, there are specially designed fine instruments and cuticle retractors (the majority of these are stick retractors made of orangewood; however, some are made of metal).

Note: These instruments must be used extremely delicately and with great care. Incorrect use may cause mechanical damage to the nail structure, and produce permanent deformation. If the instruments are not adequately sterilized before use, there is a risk of introducing bacterial or fungal infection into the nail. In any case, such manipulations should only be done by someone experienced. Many dermatologists in fact are against any unnecessary manipulations in the area of the cuticle, and advise against cuticle 'retractors' – even those made of orangewood. If the manicure requires attention to the cuticles, this should be done after softening the skin by soaking and by pushing back the cuticle using a moistened cloth.

Manicure also includes the correct and proper use of cosmetic preparations for use on the nails, and which will be described below, such as nail polish, nail moisturizers, and others.

Nail polish
Nail polish is used for:

- colour – both for beautification and to cover up blemishes in the nails' colour;
- strengthening weak nails.

The main constituent of nail polishes is **nitrocellulose**, a stable substance that mechanically strengthens the nail. It is derived from plant cellulose, and is dissolved in organic solvents. Once applied to the nail, the solvents evaporate, leaving a thin film of nitrocellulose, which is hard, shiny and waterproof.

Other substances used in nail polishes, apart from nitrocellulose, include compounds based on **vinyl**, **methylacrylate** and **cellulose acetate**. However, these compounds cannot reach the toughness and surface hardness of nitrocellulose.

Other compounds in nail polishes

Nitrocellulose has several disadvantages. The thin film produced by nitrocellulose has low gloss, it is brittle and it adheres poorly to the nail plate. To overcome these drawbacks, other compounds are being added to nail polish preparations:

- **Solvents**, whose function is to keep the product in liquid form for long periods, and prevent it from drying out. The most commonly used solvents are alkyl esters, glycol ethers and alcohols.
- **Resins**, which improve the adhesion of the product to the nail. They also give the polish its characteristic glossy appearance.
- **Plasticizers**, which are chemical flexibilizers. They provide flexibility and softness to the nail and the nail becomes less brittle. Plasticizers may also improve adhesion and gloss. The common plasticizers in the cosmetic industry are dibutyl phthalate, camphor and castor oil.
- **Colouring agents** give the nail plate the desired colour. Guanine, derived from scales of Atlantic herring, produces a pearlescent shade. Bismuth oxychloride and mica coated with titanium dioxide impart to the nail an iridescent appearance.
- Some nail polishes contain **nylon fibres**, to thicken and strengthen the nail.
- Some nail polishes contain **proteins**, **gelatin** and various **vitamins**.
- Some nail polish preparations contain tiny **pellets**, often made of nickel (and sometimes of **copper**) to help in mixing the polish before use. Most of them are now coated to prevent possible allergic reactions in those who are allergic to copper or nickel.

Application of nail polish

Nail polish should be applied evenly over the nail surface. Care should be taken to prevent it from getting on the skin folds and the areas around the nails. Ideally, it should be applied from the base of the nail towards the edge. If too much nail polish has been applied and it has got onto the areas around the nail, the excess should be carefully wiped off with a cotton applicator soaked in nail polish remover.

Undesirable side-effects of nail polish

Prolonged use of dark-coloured nail polishes can eventually lead to changes in **colour** and **staining** of the nails. As the colouring agents in the nail polish permeate the nail plate, their colour changes from the original shade of the nail polish; for example, a nail polish that was originally red usually stains the nail orange-yellow. With time, of course, the problem resolves as the nail grows out. To some extent, this problem can be avoided by applying a colourless base coating to the nail before the nail polish itself.

Allergic reactions can take the form of redness, burning, itching, sensitivity or swelling. The reaction may not be limited to the area immediately around the nail. In fact, **local** reactions to nail polish are rare. On the other hand, since the fingers come into contact with other areas of the body (for example, while scratching the nose or rubbing the eyes), allergic reactions may appear in these areas fairly frequently. Hence, skin inflammation may appear on the eyelids, on various parts of the face, or on the genitalia as a result of using nail polish. If this sort of reaction occurs, a dermatologist should be consulted. There are tests that can be done to identify the specific component of the nail polish that caused the reaction.

Nail hardeners

The purpose of nail hardeners is to harden brittle nails. In fact, nail hardeners are a variant of nail polish, except that they are clear, with no coloured additives. They also have a slightly different composition. Substances likely to be present in nail hardeners include acrylate polymers, and a mixture of proteins and salts of various metals. Gelatin has the reputation of being useful as a nail hardener, but its true effectiveness is controversial.

- Some nail hardeners contain **formaldehyde**. In high concentrations, formaldehyde can cause serious side-effects and damage to the nail structure. In the USA and most European countries, nail hardeners that contain more than 5% formaldehyde are prohibited. In addition, while using nail hardeners, one should use nail shields that protect the skin around the nail plate. In recent years, formaldehyde has been replaced by other substances, such as polyesters, polyamides and acrylate polymers.
- Some nail hardeners contain **nylon fibres**, which harden the nail plate even further.

In general, nail hardener should be applied only to the outer edges of the nails; it is that part of the nail which is most likely to split or break, and there is no sense in covering the entire nail plate with hardener. Also, as with nail polish, care should be taken to avoid getting the nail hardener on the areas around the nail or on the nail fold.

Nail moisturizers

The purpose of these products is to add moisture to the nail plate. They usually contain proteins, fatty acids, lanolin and amino acids. Newer products contain vitamins and various plant extracts. Moisturizers are applied to the nail with a brush or by massaging them into the nail.

Nail polish removers

The most commonly used solvent for removal of nail products is **acetone**. Other solvents are based on alcohols. Some also contain fatty compounds such as lanolin, which are said to produce an impermeable layer on the nail in order to increase the moisture content of the nail.

Nail polish should be removed using paper tissue or cotton wool, by repeatedly rubbing in the remover.

Side-effects of nail polish remover

These products can cause the nail plate to dry out, and can cause irritation of the surrounding tissues. Drying out of the nail can lead to nail brittleness.

To avoid these problems:

- Nail polish remover should not be used too frequently – no more than once a week.
- Removers containing fats, which lessen the drying effect, should be used.
- The hands should be washed thoroughly after using polish remover.

Note: Nail polish removers are basically poisonous, and inhaling of the fumes could be dangerous.

Artificial nails

It is not uncommon for artificial nails to cause undesirable side-effects. The possibility of these side-effects should be considered before using artificial nails. If artificial nails are used to hide defects in the natural nails, it is advisable to obtain a dermatologist's opinion first. Often there is an effective medical treatment for a deformity of the nails. Furthermore, in these cases, not only may the artificial nails be ineffective, they may even aggravate the situation.

Nail tips
These are popular because they are easy to use. They are produced in a variety of shapes, sizes and colours. The nail tips are glued on using **acrylic glue**. They are usually made of nylon or plastic. These compounds do not cause allergic reactions. However, the acrylic glue can cause skin irritation and allergic reactions. Furthermore, using nail tips can lead to excessive brittleness of the natural nails, to splitting, and to changes in their colour. A stronger glue is based on **ethyl 2-cyanoacrylate**, which provides better adhesion, but can cause damage and disfigurement to the natural nail.

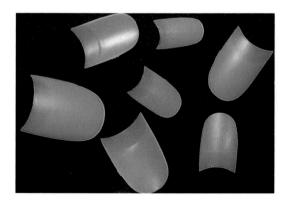

Preformed plastic nail tips.

Nail tips should not be left on for more than a few hours at a time (up to a maximum of 18 hours a day). They must be removed before retiring to bed. Covering up and 'sealing off' the natural nail for prolonged periods with nail tips may cause degenerative changes or fungal infections in the natural nail.

It should also be remembered that removing the glued-on nail tips without taking due care may result in pulling off some layers of the natural nail. The nail tips must be removed carefully and delicately, using a fatty nail polish remover.

Nail tips are often used as extensions of sculptured nails. Professional nail technicians usually coat these tips with artificial nail products to create longer-lasting nail extensions. Most nail technicians feel it is too time-consuming to sculpt nails, and these tips speed the process.

Nail sculpturing

This method is intended to achieve a stronger, longer, more attractive nail, which can be built up to any desired length. The sculpturing is achieved by using **acrylic polymers** that are built on to a metal form attached to the existing nail plate, as will be described below. Nail sculpturing is usually carried out in cosmetic offices, but there are kits for home use. The result is quite appealing and aesthetically pleasing, especially if the underlying nail was deformed or disfigured. The sculptured nail is an almost perfect continuation of the natural nail, and is almost impossible to distinguish from it.

Method of nail sculpturing

1 The nail is cleaned.
2 The nail is abraded with a nail file or a pumice stone to clean the plate more thoroughly and remove leftover cosmetics (e.g. nail polish) that have adhered to it. In addition, this roughens the nail's surface, which improves adhesion of the sculptured nail.
3 Some dermatologists suggest the application of antibacterial and antifungal solutions to the surface, to prevent bacterial or fungal infection.

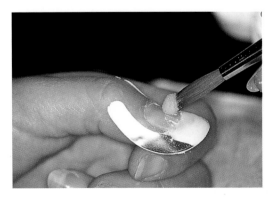

Metallized paper board template for nail sculpturing.

4 A flexible template is inserted under the natural nail plate, on top of which the nail will be built.
5 The sculptured nail is made by applying layers of acrylic polymers onto the surface of the natural nail with a brush. The polymers can then be shaped into the desired length and width.

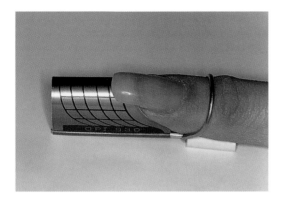

Teflon template for nail sculpturing.

The acrylic material on top of the nail plate is clear, but over the free edges of the nail it looks opaque. This appearance mimics the natural appearance of a nail closely.

Sculptured nails can be removed with nail polish remover. Light-cured gels are resistant to solvents, and where these have been used, the nail should be removed slowly with a medium-grit file (not a drill).

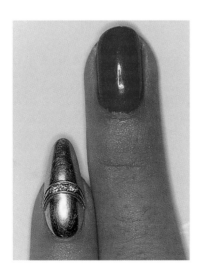

Preformed nail in gold plate.

Undesirable side-effects of artificial nails

Prolonged use of any type of artificial nail can damage the natural nails. Artificial nails cover the natural nail, and do not allow the various substances that accumulate under them to evaporate. This may result in softening of the natural nail, with the appearance of **onychodystrophy** – deformation of the nail.

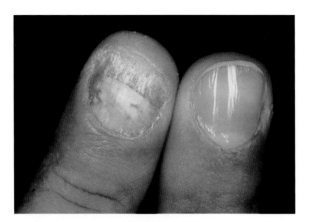

Onychodystrophy (left) following nail sculpturing.

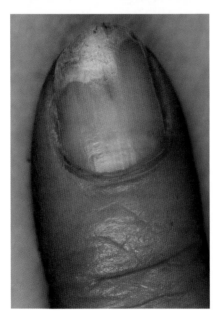

Onycholysis.

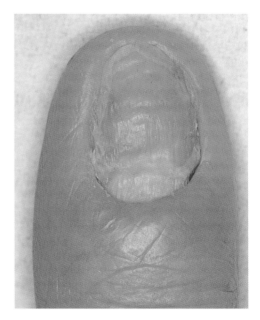

Mild paronychia: note the redness and swelling of tissues around the nail plate.

With sculptured nails, since the adhesion between the artificial nail and the natural nail is stronger than that between the natural nail and the nail bed, a condition known as **onycholysis** can occur, in which the nail plate lifts off from the nail bed. The white appearance of the nail plate in onycholysis is due to this separation of the nail from its bed.

There may be allergic reactions to one of the components of the substances used to build up the artificial nail. These reactions usually appear about two or four months after nail sculpturing. Sometimes the reaction occurs later – even after a year. The first sign of an allergic reaction is usually itching of the nail bed.

The use of artificial nails can also lead to a condition known as **paronychia** – a bacterial infection of the tissues around the nail.

Rarely, the whole of the natural nail is lost as a result of using artificial nails.

Some concluding comments regarding artificial nails
- It is best not to use them, if possible.
- If a patient wants artificial nails because of an unsightly appearance of the natural nails, a dermatologist's opinion should be sought before using artificial nails. It is possible that the problem can be solved medically.
- Whatever type of artificial nails is used, they should be removed as soon as possible.
- If side-effects occur, the artificial nails should be removed immediately using nail polish remover, or with a medium-grit file if light-cured gels have been used.

Appendix 1

What method should one use to apply cosmetic preparations to the face and neck?

In various books on cosmetics one finds illustrations and pictures meant to instruct one how to correctly apply emulsions, creams and ointments to the face and neck area.

What is the preferred method for topical applications?

This question was asked regarding the application of moisturizing preparations and sunscreens, and also in regard to creams and cleansing emulsions, for cleaning and disinfecting of the facial skin by cosmeticians.

Many dermatologists feel that there is no significance to the direction or way in which the preparations are applied (in straight or circular motions). However, most dermatologists agree that it is important that the application be done gently in order to avoid repeated, unnecessary stretching of the skin. Other dermatologists may tend to be pedantic about the methods they recommend for applying cosmetic preparations to the facial skin:

- Applying the preparation from the centre of the face and outwards is easier and simpler.
- It is preferable that the preparation be applied parallel to the natural skin lines of the face and neck (see below), and not perpendicular to them. In this way, one avoids repeated stretching of the skin in a way that later encourages the appearance of wrinkles.

Therefore, according to the above stated principles, the preferable directions for applying preparations to the skin are as illustrated below:

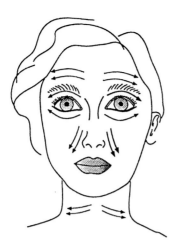

Preferable directions of application.

What are natural skin lines?

Natural skin lines are created according to how the collagen fibres are arranged. The directions in which facial muscles are used determine the direction of the natural skin lines. Later in life, these skin lines appear as skin wrinkles.

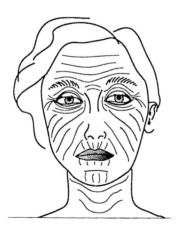

Later in life, natural skin lines appear as skin wrinkles.

As mentioned above, cosmetic preparations should be applied as gently as possible, parallel to the natural skin lines and in the direction of the face and neck wrinkles.

Appendix 2
Glossary

Acne A disease of the hair follicles and associated sebaceous glands. The onset of acne is frequently related to hormonal changes that occur during adolescence.

Acnegenic An acnegenic substance is one that may cause a skin reaction resulting in acne in the area of its application. In that case the acne is characterized by pustular lesions (containing pus) that appear one to two weeks after using the substance. Certain cosmetic preparations may contain acnegenic substances.

Acute An acute illness is one that develops rapidly and that is not prolonged; it either resolves or progresses to a chronic phase.

Allantoin A substance in wide use in cosmetics. In the past, it was extracted from various plants; nowadays it is mainly synthesized from uric acid. It is said to have 'soothing' properties on the skin, and the ability to heal wounds. It is a common ingredient of moisturizing preparations and products designed to soothe irritated skin.

Allergy A state of excessive sensitivity resulting from an immunological response of the body to some substance. Allergy can occur following inhalation of the offending substance, from swallowing it, or from direct contact of the substance with the skin.

Aloe vera This plant extract is said to have 'soothing' properties. It is present in a wide range of cosmetics, and also in home medications for use in mild burns, wounds and various skin inflammations.

Alpha-hydroxy acids Substances derived from vegetable and fruit extracts. Preparations containing alpha-hydroxy acids may have a beneficial effect on skin ageing, particularly those processes due to excessive sun exposure. Alpha-hydroxy acids also bleach various pigmented lesions of the skin. In low concentrations, they function as effective moisturizing agents.

Anagen The stage of active hair growth, when the hair cells are dividing, and the hair is growing.

Antibacterial A substance that kills or inhibits the growth of bacteria.

Antibiotics Substances that kill or inhibit the growth of bacteria. Antibiotics are produced from certain bacteria or moulds.

Antimicrobial A substance that kills or inhibits the growth of bacteria or other microorganisms.

Antiperspirants Preparations that reduce sweating, which are usually made up of aluminium compounds. These substances penetrate the duct of the sweat gland, block it, and thereby reduce the secretion of sweat.

Antiseptic A substance that kills or inhibits the growth of bacteria or other microorganisms, usually applied to body surfaces or used to disinfect medical equipment.

Apocrine sweat gland Specialized sweat gland present in the axillae (armpits) and groin. The fluid secreted by apocrine glands is relatively thick, and contains various organic compounds. These organic substances are broken down by bacteria, giving rise to an unpleasant body odour.

Aromatic oils Oily substances derived from various plants, which are volatile liquids with characteristic fragrances. These oils are reputed to have anti-inflammatory and antibacterial properties, as well as a cooling, soothing effect on the skin. They are found in a wide range of cosmetic preparations, including cleansing preparations (soaps and shampoos).

Arrector pilorum muscle A tiny muscle attached to a hair. When this muscle contracts, the hair stands up straight. The sudden contraction of these muscles creates 'goose bumps'.

Astringents Preparations that in essence impart a feeling of coolness and freshness to the skin. The skin feels 'taut', and the skin pores are temporarily constricted. Astringents contain a mixture of alcohol and water, aluminium or zinc salts, and other components such as menthol, camphor and plant extracts (such as witch hazel).

Atopic dermatitis A skin disease characterized by dryness, redness and severe itching. This disease is one of the group of conditions known as atopic diseases. Asthma and allergic rhinitis (hay fever) are also included in this group.

Atrophy In general, this term refers to a decrease in size or wasting of a tissue or organ. Atrophic skin is thin and delicate. Severely atrophic skin wrinkles like cigarette paper, and becomes transparent, so that the underlying blood vessels become visible through it. Skin becomes atrophic with age. The prolonged use of corticosteroid-containing preparations on the skin can make it atrophic.

Azelaic acid A substance used in the treatment of acne. It is also used for lightening dark skin lesions.

Bacterium A single-celled microorganism, often referred to as a 'germ'. Bacteria cannot be seen with the naked eye, but can be seen with a light microscope. Of the many types of bacteria in nature, most are not harmful to humans. A small number of bacteria are capable of causing infections in humans (e.g. pneumonia, tonsillitis, cellulitis, etc.)

Benzoyl peroxide An oxidizing substance that attacks bacteria, it is useful in the treatment of acne and is present in many acne preparations, including creams, emulsions, soaps and others.

Biopsy Removal of a piece of tissue from the body (e.g. a piece of skin) for the purpose of microscopic and laboratory examination.

Calamine A mixture of zinc oxide with a small amount of iron oxide; it has a soothing effect on the skin, and decreases itching.

Cancer A malignant growth or tumor.

Carcinoma This term embraces a wide range of malignant growths of various types. Common skin growths that are carcinomas are basal cell carcinoma and squamous cell carcinoma.

Catagen A stage in the life cycle of hair. It is a brief (about two weeks) transitory phase, when the hair stops growing and the cells at its base start to degenerate.

Cationic surfactants A group of surfactants that are used in shampoos and hair conditioners because of their ability to neutralize the negative electric charges on the surface of the hair (see **Surfactants**).

'Cellulite' A lay term (unrelated to any medical term) describing an unattractive distribution of subcutaneous fat in the body, especially in the thighs and buttocks.

Ceramides These compose approximately 40% of the fatty acids within cells. They play an important role in maintaining the keratin layer of the skin. Recently ceramides have been increasingly used in the cosmetics industry, both as moisturizing agents and as protective agents for the prevention and repair of damage caused by exposure to various chemicals.

Chloasma See **Melasma**.

Chronic A chronic disease is one that exists for a prolonged period.

Cleansing cream Creams containing cleansing substances (see **Surfactants**), designed to clean the face. They are meant to stay on the face for a short time only, and are then wiped off with a tissue or moist cloth, or rinsed off with water.

Cold cream A cream that gives a feeling of coolness when applied to the skin. It is made up of a simple mixture of oil and water. When applied to the skin, the water separates out from the oil, and quickly evaporates from the surface of the skin. This process of evaporation produces a cold feeling on the skin (hence the name of this cream).

Collagen A protein present in the dermis. Collagen is arranged in the form of intertwined fibres, which give the skin strength and resilience.

Comedogenic A comedogenic substance is one that is an ingredient of a cosmetic preparation for application to the skin, and which is liable to cause acne. In that case, the acne is characterized by the appearance of **comedones**.

Comedone The basic lesion in acne, resulting from the accumulation of compressed keratin and fat in a hair follicle. An **open comedone** (blackhead) results when the opening of the hair follicle is widened by the material that builds up inside the follicle. A **closed comedone** (whitehead) occurs when the opening of the follicle remains closed.

Conditioners (hair) Substances that produce a layer that coats the hair, and gives the hair a smooth and uniform look. Conditioners neutralize the electric charges on the surface of the hair, making it easier to comb and manage.

Contact dermatitis Skin inflammation resulting from direct skin contact with various substances. Contact dermatitis may occur by means of a direct mechanism (when it is called **irritant dermatitis**), or via an allergic mechanism (in **allergic contact dermatitis**).

Cortex (of the hair) The central layer seen in a cross-section of a hair. The cortex is made up of cells that are degenerating and dying as they move up the hair, to the skin surface.

Corticosteroids A general name for a group of hormones that are produced naturally in the body. Some corticosteroids have anti-inflammatory properties. Hence these substances are widely used in dermatology against inflammatory diseases of the skin. Prolonged and excessive use of corticosteroids, whether taken by mouth or by application to the skin, may result in serious side-effects. Always consult a physician before using any preparation that contains corticosteroids.

Cosmetician Someone involved in the field of cosmetics, which is directed towards the care, protection, and improvement of the appearance of the skin.

Cosmetics A wide field related to the various aspects of appearance and beauty. It mainly involves the care, protection, and improvement of the appearance of the skin. The origin of the word is from the Greek *kosmos*, meaning 'order'.

Cosmetologist Someone who is an expert in the research aspects of cosmetics, and who may be a chemist, a biologist or a physician. This definition varies from one country to another. In some countries, such as in the USA, it is a formal title subjected to the regulations of each state, for which one has to graduate from a school of cosmetics. In other countries, cosmetology is not a formally recognized degree.

Cosmetology A general term covering the research aspects of cosmetics, embracing biological, chemical and medical aspects.

Couperose An alternative term for **telangiectasis**.

Cream A semi-solid **emulsion**. Creams, obtained from a combination of a fatty substance with water, are common bases in cosmetics and dermatology, and may contain many different cosmetic and medical substances.

Cuticle (hair) The outermost layer of the hair shaft, which is made up of a layer of individual cells, overlapping each other. The cuticle acts as the protective layer of the hair.

Cuticle (nail) The skin fold at the base of the nail.

Cyst A fluid-filled cavity in the skin. Cysts may occur in acne.

Dandruff (scales) Fragments of keratin that are shed from the skin surface as part of the process of epidermal cell turnover. So long as the rate of cell turnover is normal, one cannot normally see these flakes. If the cell turnover is increased, more and more dead flakes of keratin appear, which may join together into larger, visible pieces, and can be seen as they come away from the scalp.

Deodorants Substances designed to prevent unpleasant body odour. Deodorants contain various combinations of antibacterial substances (substances active against bacteria), substances that adsorb odours, and substances that mask odours.

Depilation A technique for removal of hair, in which the removal is superficial, and takes place at or near the skin surface – in contrast to **epilation** it does not involve the hair root. Depilation can be carried out, for example, by shaving or by using depilatory creams. Regardless of the method used, depilation is only of temporary value.

Dermatitis A term used for **inflammation** of the skin.

Dermatologist A 'skin doctor'; a physician who deals with the various aspects of skin diseases.

Dermatology The field of medicine dealing with the diagnosis and treatment of skin diseases.

Dermis A layer of the skin, containing collagen and elastin fibres. The dermis also contains blood vessels, nerves, sensory organs, sebaceous glands, sweat glands and hair follicles.

Dihydroxyacetone A substance present in artificial tanning preparations. Dihydroxyacetone reacts chemically with proteins in the outer (dead keratin) layer of the epidermis. In so doing, it imparts an artificial, brown to yellow suntan-like colour to the skin, which lasts for about three to five days.

Eccrine sweat glands These are scattered all over the body. The sweat secreted by eccrine glands plays an important role in regulating body temperature. This sweat does *not* cause body odour.

Elastin A protein present in the dermis. It is arranged in fibres, and gives the skin its elastic characteristics, so that when it is stretched, it falls back into place.

Electrolysis A method of permanent hair removal, carried out by inserting a fine metal needle into the opening of the hair follicle. An electric current is then passed through the needle, which may destroy the active cells at the hair root.

EMLA (Eutectic Mixture of Lidocaine and Prilocaine) Contains local anaesthetic agents. It is used before performing painful procedures on the skin (such as removal of hair with an electric needle). EMLA should be applied to the skin some 60 minutes prior to performing the procedure, and an occlusive dressing placed over it. It lessens the pain that may accompany the course of various medical/cosmetic procedures performed on the skin.

Emulsifier (also called an '**emulsifying agent**') A substance (natural or synthetic) that separates oil from water. In that way, it stabilizes emulsions (which contain oil and water), so that the oil droplets remain dispersed throughout the water as a homogeneous mixture. In the absence of an emulsifier, an oil–water mixture will separate into two distinct layers.

Emulsion A mixture of oil and water. An emulsion is a basic preparation that may incorporate many cosmetic substances or medications. If it contains a relatively large proportion of water, it is more liquid (and is then known as a **liquid emulsion**). If the preparation does not contain a lot of water its texture is not liquid, but rather semi-solid. In that case the substance is a **cream**.

Epidermis The outermost layer of the skin. At the base of this layer, new cells are constantly and steadily formed by a process of cell division.

Epilation A technique for the removal of hair that involves removing the hair together with its root. The removal of hair by epilation may be temporary (e.g. by pulling out the hair), or permanent (e.g. by using an electric needle).

Erythema Redness of the skin. There may be many reasons for the skin becoming red, for example in certain diseases, or following sun exposure.

Esthetician Someone involved in the field of cosmetics, which is directed towards the care, protection, and improving the appearance of the skin.

Eumelanin A pigment that is similar in its chemical structure to melanin. It gives the hair a brown–black colour.

Fibroblast A cell in the dermis of the skin that is responsible for producing the intercellular matrix and collagen fibres.

Folliculitis Inflammation of a hair follicle. The word is made up of *follicle*, and *-itis*, which is a standard suffix in medical terminology meaning 'inflammation'. Folliculitis can occur, for instance, after shaving, after plucking hair or after use of an electric needle – as the result of microscopic injuries that occur to the follicle during the shaving or plucking process.

Foundation cream In essence, a foundation cream is a moisturizing cream. In many cases, it contains a sunscreen. Apart from maintaining the skin's moisture, and protecting it from the sun, foundation cream gives the face a smooth, uniform appearance, and conceals skin lesions.

Gamma-linoleic acid A fatty acid that is said to have anti-inflammatory properties. It also serves as an occlusive substance in the keratin layer of the skin, thereby contributing to the defensive properties of skin.

Gel A common base used in cosmetics and dermatology. Gels may contain a wide range of active ingredients or medications. A gel is similar to a cream in its consistency, but contains less fat; it is therefore used on skin that tends to be oily.

Hair follicle An elongated tube-like depression in the skin from which a hair grows.

Hamamelis See **Witch hazel**.

Horny layer See **Keratin layer**.

Humectants Substances that are effective at absorbing water, and commonly used in moisturizing substances. Some humectants (e.g. urea or lactic acid) can penetrate the keratin layer of the skin and increase its moisture content.

Hyaluronic acid A component of the intercellular substance in the dermis. It absorbs water efficiently, and is commonly used in moisturizing compounds.

Hydrogen peroxide A strong antiseptic liquid. Hydrogen peroxide is not used as a routine antiseptic for wounds, etc., since it also damages normal body tissues. Its use is limited to especially contaminated, infected wounds, such as bites. Hydrogen peroxide is also used for bleaching hair.

Hydroquinone A substance used for lightening dark skin lesions (such as 'pregnancy mask' or 'sun spots').

Hypoallergenic A preparation that ostensibly does not contain substances that tend to cause skin irritation or allergic reactions (mainly perfumes and various preservatives). However, even hypoallergenic preparations may cause skin irritation or allergy.

Inflammation A defensive response of the body to certain processes, including various infections and other insults. The signs of inflammation are localized warmth (in the area involved), redness, swelling, and sometimes pain and loss of function of the inflamed organ.

Iodine An active substance that inhibits and kills bacteria and other microorganisms. Iodine can appear in different forms in various preparations, e.g. tincture of iodine (a preparation based on iodine dissolved in alcohol) and povidone iodine (a compound containing iodine with a polymer that ensures the slow release of the iodine).

Isotretinoin The commercial name for a medication from the retinoid group of compounds, substances that are chemically similar to vitamin A. It is used in the treatment of acne. It may only be given on the recommendation of a dermatologist.

Keratin This protein, the major component of the keratin layer of the skin, is also present in hair and nails. Keratin gives the skin its strength and provides protection from external insults.

Keratin (horny) layer The outermost layer of the skin. It is made up of flat, dead cells lying one on top of the other. As new cells are formed in the skin, the outer dead cells are pushed out, directed to the surface of the skin and are shed from the skin.

Keratinocytes The cells that make up the epidermis. They are also known as squamous cells (Latin *squama* = a scale).

Keratolytic A keratolytic substance is one that can dissolve and remove keratin from the skin. Keratolytic preparations are used for treating areas of thickened skin. Sometimes, in the treatment of acne, keratolytic preparations are used to remove the keratin that occludes the opening of the hair follicle.

Keratosis An abnormal situation characterized by localized or generalized thickening of the keratin layer of the skin. It may appear as part of a cancerous or precancerous process (such as solar keratosis) or various inflammatory processes.

Langerhans Langerhans cells are cells in the skin related to the immune system.

Lanolin A fatty substance that is a complex mixture, derived from sheep's wool. Lanolin is a common ingredient of moisturizing substances.

Liposomes Microscopic spheres made up of **phospholipids**. Recently they have become widely used in dermatology and the cosmetics industry. The aim is to introduce medications and various cosmetic substances into liposomes, so they (the liposomes) act as a carrier to help the active ingredient that is inside them penetrate the skin.

Liquid emulsion An emulsion that appears in the form of a liquid, derived from a mixture of water and oil (**emulsion**). A liquid emulsion is a base that may contain many cosmetic or medicinal ingredients.

Lotion The simple definition of a lotion is a preparation that contains liquid components. However, the more accurate, scientific definition of lotion is a mixture of oil, powder and water.

Lunula The pale, crescent-like structure that is found at the base of the nail. The outer part of the nail matrix (the area from which the nail grows) lies under this region.

Malignant melanoma A malignant skin tumour. The mortality rate from malignant melanoma is high, and it is therefore extremely important to detect this lesion early, and remove it in its entirety. Malignant melanoma arises from **melanocytes** in the skin.

Manicure A term that covers numerous procedures involved in the care of the fingernails. The word is derived from the Latin *manus* = hand, *curo* = to care for.

Medulla (of the hair) The inner layer seen in a cross-section of a hair. Sometimes it is missing, and sometimes it is not continuous along the length of a hair. The absence or presence of the medulla can affect the sheen and shade of the hair.

Melanin A pigment produced by melanocytes in the skin. Melanin gives the skin a dark colour, and it plays a role in the skin's protection against the sun.

Melanocytes Cells in the epidermis that produce **melanin**.

Melanocytic naevus This is the lesion commonly known as a mole, or as a 'beauty spot'. It originates from melanocytes – the cells that produce melanin. Melanin is the pigment that gives the skin its dark colour.

Melasma (Chloasma) 'Pregnancy mask'. A specific distribution of pigment on the face, seen in some women. This phenomenon develops more commonly during pregnancy. In melasma, there are light or dark brown areas on the upper lip, the forehead and chin, usually symmetrical. There is presumably a hormonal basis for this phenomenon.

Metastases Groups of malignant cells that break away from the primary cancerous tumor and find their way to other areas of the body. In those areas, the metastatic cells continue to multiply uncontrollably and destroy the surrounding tissues.

Micelle The soap structure that surrounds fat and dirt particles, enabling them to be removed from the skin by rinsing with water.

Moisturizing cream Designed to increase the moisture content of the skin. Moisturizing creams contain occlusive fatty substances, or water-absorbent substances.

Nail bed The soft skin underneath the nail plate.

Nail matrix The living, growing part of the nail, under the nail base. The cells of the nail matrix are continuously, steadily dividing, and in that way the nail grows.

Nail plate The external, visible part of the nail.

Neoplasm (Also called **Tumour** or **Cancer**) A lesion arising from the uncontrolled growth of some tissue in the body. If the growth is benign, it remains confined to the area of the body from where it arose; a malignant tumour, on the other hand, tends to spread aggressively to nearby tissues, and to more distant tissues in the body.

Night cream Night creams are also called 'nourishing creams'. They have a very high fat content, and are supposed to contain various ingredients that penetrate the skin. For that to occur, the cream has to stay on the skin for several hours. Therefore these creams are applied at night, before going to bed. The 'nourishing' components of these creams consist of various active ingredients, which are believed by some to benefit the skin after they penetrate deeply into it.

Nitrocellulose The main ingredient in nail polish and nail hardeners. It is a very stable substance that provides the nail with mechanical strength. Once the nail polish has been applied, various solvents that it contains evaporate, leaving the nitrocellulose behind as a thin, hard, shiny, waterproof layer on the nail.

NMF (Natural Moisturizing Factor) A mixture of substances present in the skin that make up approximately 20–25% of the keratin layer. This mixture is able to retain the moisture content of the keratin layer.

Nodule An inflammatory lump in the skin. Compared with a papule, a nodule is deeper in the skin. The distinction between a nodule and a papule is based on how they feel to the touch. Nodules may appear in a wide range of diseases and abnormalities of the skin. Acne may be characterized by the appearance of nodules.

Onychodystrophy Distortion of the shape of the nail.

Onycholysis This is when the **nail plate** comes away from the **nail bed**. When that happens, white areas appear on the nail plate.

Organic In the biological sciences, an organic substance is usually said to be one derived from living matter; in chemistry, an organic compound is one that contains carbon atoms.

Oxygen free radicals These are byproducts of chemical processes that oxygen molecules undergo. They are normally produced regularly and naturally in many body tissues, but certain factors (e.g. solar radiation, smoking, environmental pollutants, and others) increase their rate of production. Oxygen free radicals can damage various body tissues. It appears that they may be involved in the development of some heart diseases, diseases of the blood vessels, and various malignant diseases. Researchers maintain that free radicals have a cumulative effect that accelerates ageing of various body tissues.

Panthenol Also known as provitamin B_5. It is said to help in wound healing and alleviating skin inflammation. It is a common ingredient in preparations used in the treatment of diaper rash in infants.

Papule A lesion of about 0.5 cm diameter that is raised above the surface of the skin. The papules seen in acne are typically pink/red in colour because of the inflammatory process.

Paraffin Paraffins are a group of fatty compounds derived from the refining of crude oil. After purification and bleaching, they are common ingredients of moisturizing agents. Paraffins may appear as liquids, semi-solids (as petroleum jelly), or solids (paraffin wax).

Paraphenylenediamine A component of permanent hair dyes.

Paronychia Infection of the tissues around the nail.

Paste A mixture of powder and an ointment. Because of its fat content, a paste has good occlusive and skin-protective properties. The powder within the paste effectively absorbs liquids. The main use of pastes is in protecting infants' skin from urine and faeces in the diaper region.

Patch test A skin test to help identify causes of skin inflammation or contact allergy. The test is carried out by using small discs containing various substances, which are attached to the patient's skin. The skin reaction is examined under each disc after 48–96 hours.

Pedicure A term that covers numerous procedures involved in the care of the foot and the toenails. The word is derived from the Latin *pedis* = foot, *curo* = to care for.

Peeling A technique for removing the outermost layer of the skin by creating a chemical burn. As the burn heals, a new outer layer of skin forms, which is smoother, tauter, more uniform and pinker than the original surface.

Permanent waving of hair Setting the hair in the form of curls. Permanent waving is achieved by a series of chemical processes performed on the hair, involving softening the hair, fashioning into the desired shape, and finally fixing it permanently in that shape. The substances used in a permanent wave are thioglycolates or chemically related substances.

Petroleum jelly A semi-solid form of **paraffin** (white soft paraffin).

Phenol A substance used for deep skin peeling. The use of phenol requires giving the patient either intravenous analgesia (pain relief) or a general anaesthetic during the procedure. When carrying out skin peeling using phenol, the patient's cardiac (heart) status must be monitored carefully, and he/she must be given intravenous fluids to prevent possible kidney damage.

Pheomelanin A pigment that is chemically similar to melanin. It gives the hair a reddish shade.

Phospholipids Fatty compounds containing phosphorus that make up the two-layered cell walls in the body. In the cosmetics industry, **liposomes**, which are made up of phospholipids, are used to help the active ingredients of various preparations penetrate the skin.

Pigment A coloured substance, such as melanin, the more of which there is, the darker the skin looks. Makeup contains various pigments to give the user a skin shade that is different from his/her natural skin colour.

Pityrosporum ovale A microscopic yeast that is commonly present in the scalp and hair follicles. Dandruff and seborrhoeic dermatitis have been attributed to *Pityrosporum ovale*. Some of the shampoos designed to treat dandruff are formulated to act upon this microscopic yeast on the surface of the scalp.

Polymers Chemical compounds made up of long chains of many small, identical, individual units.

Psoralens A group of substances that increase the skin's sensitivity to type A ultraviolet radiation, and hence result in faster tanning. They are used in a number of skin diseases. Not only do psoralens accelerate skin tanning, but at the same time they may increase all the damaging effects of solar radiation on the skin, and are therefore prohibited for use as routine tanning agents.

Purpura Localized bleeding into the skin. Purpura occurs in various diseases – both skin diseases and general diseases. Among other things, prolonged use of corticosteroid-containing preparations can cause purpura to appear in the treated areas.

Pustules Small blisters on the skin, which contain pus.

Resorcinol A **keratolytic** substance that also possesses a degree of antiseptic effect. It is an older treatment for acne.

Retinoic acid This has a similar chemical structure to vitamin A. Preparations containing retinoic acid are used in the treatment of acne, and for bleaching dark areas of skin. Retinoic acid is also used to repair and halt ageing processes in the skin – particularly those processes related to excessive exposure to the sun.

Salicylic acid This is the active component of aspirin (the chemical name for aspirin is acetylsalicylic acid). When applied to the skin, salicylic acid is **keratolytic**, and is used to dissolve and remove excessive keratin from the skin.

Scalpel A very sharp, special knife used by surgeons.

Sebaceous glands Glands in the skin that are attached to hair follicles. They secrete their fatty product (sebum) into the hair follicle via a small secretory duct. Sebum provides a fatty layer on the surface of the skin and on the outer surface of the hair, which protects them and prevents them from getting too dry.

Seborrhoea A state characterized by excessive secretion of the sebaceous glands in the skin, producing an excess of sebum. The skin and hair look greasy. In this situation, there is usually flakiness of the skin.

Seborrhoeic dermatitis An inflammatory skin condition that occurs in areas with numerous sebaceous glands. Seborrhoeic dermatitis goes on for years, with periods of improvement and flare-ups, and is characterized by redness and the appearance of flaky scales. In adults, seborrhoeic dermatitis tends to appear mainly on the scalp, alongside the nose, and above the eyebrows.

Sebum A fatty substance secreted by the sebaceous glands, which are connected to the hair follicles. Sebum provides an oily layer that covers the skin and hair, which is protective and prevents drying out.

Skin peeling See **Peeling**.

Solar keratosis A lesion that tends to appear in fair-skinned people, above the age of 40. The lesions appear on areas exposed to the sun. They are slightly raised, dry, rough and, pink/red, with a fine, scaly surface. Solar keratoses are defined as precancerous lesions that are not considered malignant.

Spermaceti A fatty substance derived from whales. Its use is banned in the USA. Consumers who are concerned about the killing of whales should avoid using moisturizing preparations containing this substance.

SPF (Sun Protection Factor) A measurement of the efficiency of a sunscreen. The SPF is determined by measuring how long the sunscreen delays the appearance of redness in the skin when exposed to the sun.

Subcutis The fatty layer under the dermis of the skin.

Sunscreens Preparations designed to protect the skin from the sun's rays. Chemical sunscreens absorb the radiation; physical sunscreens act as a mirror and reflect the rays back from the skin.

Surfactants (surface-active agents) Water-soluble compounds that form the major ingredient of soaps and shampoos. Molecules of surfactant surround the particles of fat and dirt on the skin surface, and thereby allow them to be removed by rinsing with water.

Suspension A product that is a combination of powder and water. In this case the powder particles are not dissolved in the water, so the preparation looks turbid rather than clear and homogeneous. Before using a suspension, it must be shaken so as to produce an even distribution of the powder particles in the liquid.

Talc This is the commercial name for zinc polysilicate. It is an inert substance in the form of a powder, and is used to minimize friction and to absorb moisture. Commercial preparations containing talc also usually contain small amounts of other substances, such as zinc oxide or aluminium silicate.

Tanning The process by which the skin becomes darker following exposure to the sun. Tanning occurs because the solar radiation causes the **melanocytes** to produce melanin, which is the pigment that gives the skin its dark colour.

Telangiectasis (Telangiectasia) Dilatation (widening) of fine, superficial blood vessels (up to approximately 1 mm in diameter) on the skin surface. This phenomenon appears as the result of cumulative damage to the skin following exposure to the sun, to radiation, etc. Various diseases can also result in the appearance of telangiectases on the skin.

Telogen The resting phase in the life cycle of a hair, during which the mechanism responsible for the cellular division in the base of the follicle is inactive for several months.

Terminal hair Coarse, thick, dark hair that is readily visible.

Thioglycolates These are present in depilatory preparations. They dissolve and break down the keratinous substance of the hair, and are used for the removal of excess body hair. Thioglycolates break the sulfur bonds that bind hair fibres, and therefore they are also used for waving hair.

Tincture An alcohol-based solution.

Titanium dioxide A substance that protects against ultraviolet radiation. It is a basic ingredient in most sunscreen preparations.

Trichloroacetic acid An acid used for skin peeling.

Triclocarban An **antibacterial** substance present in various deodorants and soaps.

Triclosan An **antibacterial** substance present in various deodorants and soaps.

Ultraviolet (UV) radiation Light rays whose wavelength is beyond the visible violet light. Excessive exposure to type A or type B ultraviolet rays produces cumulative damage to the skin, which may manifest itself as 'sun spots', wrinkles and various skin tumours.

Vanishing cream A cream with a relatively high water content. Because of its 'watery' nature, it washes off readily. Since it is easier to apply, to rinse off and to wipe off the skin, it is generally used as a day cream. The advantage of using a vanishing cream is that, once it is applied to the skin, it is virtually invisible, and the thin layer on the face can hardly be seen.

Varicose veins Dilated veins that appear usually on the lower limbs; varicose veins are the result of faulty functioning of the valves in the veins.

Vellus hair Fine, thin, light hair that is hardly noticeable.

Venous insufficiency Abnormal and ineffective function of the venous blood vessels, affecting the blood flow through them.

Vitamin A compound that belongs to a family of organic substances present in tiny quantities in food, which are essential for the normal physiological function of the body.

Vitamin D A vitamin that is necessary, among other things, for building up bones and maintaining their strength. Exposure to sunlight promotes production of vitamin D in the body.

Witch hazel (Hamamelis) This plant extract is said to be able to constrict skin pores. It is a common component of astringent preparations.

Zinc pyrithione A component of many shampoos designed for treating dandruff.

Index